TOOTH FITNESS

TOOTH FITNESS

YOUR GUIDE TO HEALTHY TEETH

Thomas McGuire, D.D.S.

St. Michael's Press

McGuire, Thomas L.

    Tooth fitness: your guide to healthy teeth
      Includes index and glossary
        1. Teeth—Care and hygiene. 2. Dentistry—preventive. 3. Prevention—dental. 4. Oral health—popular works. 5. Dental care—hygiene.

Library of Congress Catalog Card Number: 93-86744

ISBN (paperback): 0-9638321-2-3

EDITOR: Alice H. Klein, Berkeley, Calif.
COVER, TEXT DESIGN, & ELECTRONIC COMPOSITION: Hal Hershey, Berkeley, Calif.
PRODUCTION COORDINATORS: Alice H. Klein and Hal Hershey
ILLUSTRATOR: Aaron Sowd, Nevada City, Calif.
PROOFREADER: David Sweet, San Francisco, Calif.
INDEXER: Do Mi Stauber, Eugene, Ore.
PHOTOGRAPHER: Sandra Fisk, San Anselmo, Calif.
BOOK MANUFACTURER: R.R. Donnelley & Sons Company, Inc.

DISCLAIMER

This book makes no medical or special claims, nor does it attempt to diagnose or treat any ailment, dental or otherwise. It does not encourage self-diagnosis for personal treatment, and the reader must take responsibility for verifying personal observations through consultation with a licensed dentist, hygienist, or medical doctor.

♲ This book is printed on recycled paper.

Manufactured in the United States of America

1 2 3 4 5 – 98 97 96 95 94

Tooth Fitness is dedicated to everyone
who has had anything to do
with making this book a reality,
but especially to my two moms,
Elizabeth Sparks and Doris Faxon.
Without them there would be no book.
They know how much I love them
and I want to publicly thank
them for everything they have done for me.
It is also dedicated to every person
who suffers from dental disease
and wants to eliminate it from their lives.

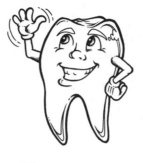

Contents

List of Technical Illustrations

Getting Started

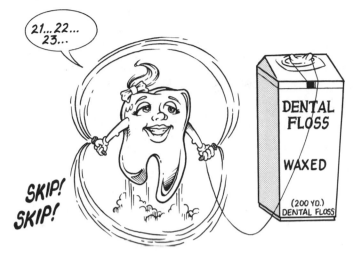

Introduction 1

For the Patient Only

Hmmmm, a book about teeth? Yep, that it is, but don't let the title throw you, because *Tooth Fitness* is about more than just teeth, their diseases, and how to keep your teeth healthy for the rest of your life. The issues I deal with go beyond how, when, and why you need to brush, floss, and irrigate. *Tooth Fitness* is also about how to survive dental experiences that can be painful, frightening, expensive, and time-consuming. It is about real choice and empowerment. Ultimately, it is about freedom and how *you* can take control of, and responsibility for, the health of your mouth.

"Well, you've got my attention, but is this book really for me?" Unfortunately, all available statistics say it is. For example, over 90 percent of the population have some form of dental disease, ranging from a little decay to severe bone loss. Less than 10 percent of those over sixty-five still have all their natural teeth, and nearly 45 percent in that age group don't have any teeth left. The American Dental Association estimates that 50 million people are fearful or anxious about dental appointments. Other sources say that as many 40 million will not see a dentist at all because of their overpowering fear. In 1994 alone, Americans will spend over $40 billion on dental repair and treatment.

As you can see, the odds are pretty good that you will eventually be found in one or more of these statistical categories (there are many more undesirable dental statistics where these came from). Below are six reasons why I think this book is for you. Once you have read through them carefully, I will be more than happy to let you be the one to decide.

☐ This book is for you especially if you already have dental disease and believe there is nothing you can do about it. That is, unless you want to continue passively accepting your fate as a helpless dental victim and wander endlessly down that rut-filled road of more decay, more fillings, more gum disease, root canals, lost teeth, bridges, and ultimately . . . those dreaded dentures.

☐ This book is for you if you're one of the millions of people who are so fearful of the dental experience that you would endure oral destruction—the tooth loss, pain, discomfort, and anxiety that so often accompany uncared for and un- 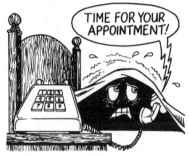 treated dental disease—rather than go to a dentist.

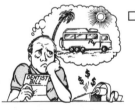 ☐ It's for you if you're one of the tens of millions who simply cannot afford the high cost of quality dentistry. It is also for you if you *can* afford it but can think of better ways to spend your money.

☐ It's for you if you're fortunate enough to have a regular dentist and hygienist but would like to improve those relationships and make your present dental experience a more productive and fulfilling one.

☐ This book is for you even if you're one of the lucky few who don't have dental disease. It's especially for you if you don't ever want to get it.

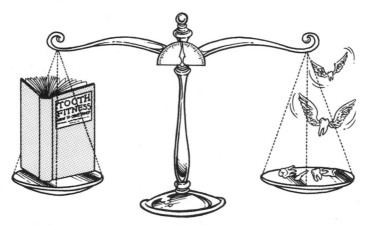

☐ And, finally, it's for you if you believe your teeth are worth the small price of this book.

Bridging the Communication Gap

Regardless of what you have been led to believe, there is absolutely no reason for you to suffer diet- and hygiene-related gum disease, decay, or tooth loss, because not only is most dental disease treatable and curable, it is also *completely preventable*. This means that you must discard the popular, but erroneous, theory that the only way to eliminate dental disease is to continue to have the damage repaired and then hope and pray the disease won't come back. So if what you've been doing hasn't worked and you want to keep your dental *past* from becoming your dental *future*, you'll need to change your dental *present*. After all, what have you got to lose . . . except your teeth!

"Well, sure," you might be thinking, "I'm all for it, but why hasn't my dentist told me how to prevent dental disease? Isn't that his responsibility?" Those are very good questions and they deserve very good answers. Today's dentist is a specialist, uniquely trained to repair the damage done by dental disease. He isn't, however, a specialist in preventive dentistry, nor was he ever trained to be one. In addition, his hands are tied by the economic realities of practicing dentistry. It is almost impossible for him to effectively teach you all you need to know while you're at the dental office and still have time to do quality repair work. This doesn't mean he doesn't care about you, your oral health, or prevention. He's doing the best he can. But the result, as I see it, is a very serious patient-dentist prevention communication gap.

In their efforts to bridge that gap, most dentists rely on auxiliary support, such as the dental hygienist and various brochures and pamphlets, to try to get across the preventive message. The problem with this approach is that the hygienist is also faced with the same economic, time, and space constraints as the dentist. If demonstrating a brushing technique and giving you a few pamphlets produced the results you were seeking there would be no problem. But although it may work for some people, for millions of others this condensed and limited approach to dental education simply does not provide all the information needed to win the war against dental disease.

A great many dentists and dental hygienists not only are aware of this communication gap but are as concerned and frustrated about it as you are. In fact, it was everyone's frustration with this problem, plus the support from hygienists and dentists, that directly led to the creation of *Tooth Fitness*. By using the book to provide you with the information you need to prevent dental disease, the dentist and hygienist can now devote their energies to the services for which they are superbly trained: repair, treatment, guidance, and support. You can then also become superbly trained: as a complete dental patient. This is a win-win situation for everyone.

The Dental Patient's Bible

More than simply a how-to book about preventive dentistry, *Tooth Fitness* is also a veritable cornucopia of important information for dealing with every aspect of your dental journey—in that sense, it's the dental patient's bible. It explains how to find the right dentist and hygienist for you, how to successfully work with them, and how to establish an effective home care program. It shows you how to overcome your dental fears and how to deal with dental emergencies. It also details how to make your child's dental trip a much better one than yours has been (that would truly be a gift to your child). It discusses AIDS and its relationship to the dental experience, explains the relationship between a healthy diet and healthy teeth, and sheds light on the fluoride and mercury controversies. And more.

Sound exciting? Well, all right, perhaps "exciting" isn't quite the right adjective when speaking of dentistry—but please don't think this is some impossible-to-understand, scientific, put-you-to-sleep dental textbook. *Tooth Fitness* is written in everyday language so that you'll actually be able to understand what I'm talking about. I don't see any reason for learning to be dull and boring. With a laugh-while-you-learn approach, your learning experience can truly be fun. But keep in mind that ultimately you will judge this book not on its literary style or its ability to entertain you, but on whether it accomplishes its aim. And its aim is to raise your dental consciousness and to produce *results*. Preventive dental education works, and even if you only take advantage of a portion of what *Tooth Fitness* offers you, it could still save you a hundred times the cost of the book in dental repair bills and time.

Remember, *prevention isn't something that is done to you, it is done by you.* The book will teach you everything you need to know to become a fully educated dental patient. But you don't have to memorize everything, and you only have to read the sections of the book that pertain to you. As part of your personal library it will always be there when you need it. Which means you don't have to try to remember every word you hear while sitting in the dental chair. You'll be able to access all this information inexpensively, at your own pace, and within the comfort of your own home. Or in your backyard, in your pool, at the beach, out on the lake, on the plane, or train, or . . .

If you want to change your dental experience from a negative one to a positive one, free yourself of dental disease, and restore your mouth to perfect health and function, you're in luck. *Tooth Fitness* will bring you a new awareness and understanding of your mouth, as well as the inner satisfaction of knowing that *if you are true to your teeth, your teeth will never be false to you.* So, my friend, read on and enjoy, for I personally guarantee that it will be an enlightening and worthwhile experience.

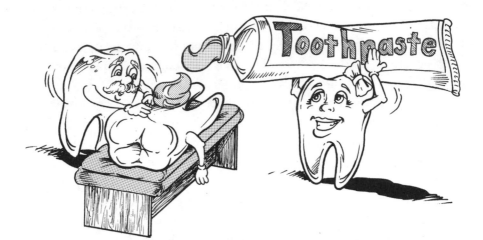

Introduction 2

For the Dentist and Dental Hygienist Only

I know that you, be you a dentist or a dental hygienist, will be exposed to *Tooth Fitness* through the media, your staff, your patients, or your peers. Though the book was written for the dental patient, the patient will not be the sole beneficiary. You, too, will benefit from it. Therefore I want to address you personally and explain why the book will be just as valuable for you and your practice as it is for your patients and their teeth.

There are many reasons, and I've listed those that I consider to be the most important.

☐ *Tooth Fitness* harmoniously bridges the communication gap between you and your patient. I have walked in your shoes and am well aware of the demands and stresses of practicing dentistry and hygiene therapy. As a dentist, specializing in preventive dentistry, I'm aware of how the economic factors of dentistry can hinder your ability to fully educate your patients. I know how difficult it is to find the time and the office space needed to furnish your patients with *all the information they need* to adequately perform their roles as patients. *Tooth Fitness* can solve the frustrating and long-standing problem of how to easily, effectively, and inexpensively educate your patients *outside* the dental office. (You may have to treat them there, but you don't have to teach them there.) The book teaches them for you and allows you to spend less time on in-office education.

☐ The book clearly defines the roles of the patient and the dental professional in the holistic preventive process. By doing so, it explains to your patients what you can do for them and why you're an indispensable part of their overall preventive program. And they'll discover, perhaps for the first time, the importance of the role they play in the healing and prevention of their disease.

As valuable as *Tooth Fitness* will be for your dental patients, however, it can't do more than help educate and motivate them by creatively providing them with information. The book makes it clear that prevention, by definition, is stopping something from taking place and that it is impossible to prevent what has already happened. They'll understand that they cannot cure and treat dental disease on their own and that no amount of brushing, flossing, water picking, hoping, or praying will ever remove calculus, fill a decayed tooth, or replace a lost one. They'll see that it is only after the mouth is restored to health that their prevention practices will be effective. And they will finally understand why it is to their functional and financial advantage to get the very best treatment available. The book will also reach those tens of millions of patients who don't now have a regular dentist and motivate them to have their teeth repaired.

Thus, with regard to preventive education, you'll be able to support your patients by becoming the *hands, eyes, ears,* and *voice* of the book. This is an invaluable role. I call this innovative and mutually supportive system Interactive Dental Prevention: the patient, dentist, and hygienist working together for the same goals.

☐ *Tooth Fitness* doesn't try to make the patient an expert on dentistry, diagnosis, or in-office treatment.

☐ It doesn't try to tell you what type of program is best for your office, how to run it, or how to treat each individual patient.

☐ Lastly, since *Tooth Fitness's* primary purpose is to educate the patient and improve dentist-patient communication, it is designed to be easily inserted into, and provide tremendous support for, any preventive program you may be using now. The philosophy behind this book is that your patients should have easy access to information about the basics of prevention. And this information should be available to them from *one source* that they can turn to as the need arises. *Tooth Fitness* is that source. We cannot realistically expect patients to gather this knowledge from scattered sources like magazine and newspaper articles that may or may not be available. Nor should they need to take up valuable time asking you questions when many of the answers can be found in this book.

There are other advantages to putting *Tooth Fitness* in your waiting room and providing copies for your patients. Soon every patient will recognize that you're not concerned only with treating and repairing dental disease. The patient will recognize that your approach is more broad based, more holistic, and that you are concerned about treating the whole person and not just a few teeth, a jawbone, or a wallet. He or she will see that you support total preventive dental education and that you're willing to back up your beliefs with action. Written by a dentist, and having the patient's interest at heart, *Tooth Fitness* will also do much toward improving our profession's tarnished image in the eyes of the public. I feel confident that once you've read it, it will become the cornerstone of your existing preventive program.

Because each dental office is unique, you will develop your own way of incorporating the book into your program. I encourage you to be creative, and I would appreciate hearing about the approach you use and how it works for you and your patients. If you have any suggestions as to how to make the book better for you and your patients, I'd like to hear those too. My simple suggestion is to make the book available to your patients, support their dental care efforts, and continue your present preventive education program. In no way is *Tooth Fitness* intended to replace what you're doing now, but I guarantee that it will make your existing program much easier, more effective, and more rewarding.

Educating our patients provides a much-needed service to our fellow human beings. Although it isn't our responsibility to force our patients to practice what we suggest, *it is our obligation to provide them with the information they need to make that choice for themselves.* *Tooth Fitness* fulfills that obligation.

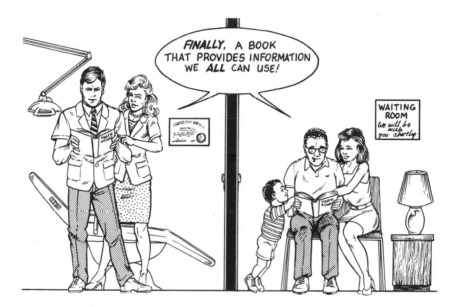

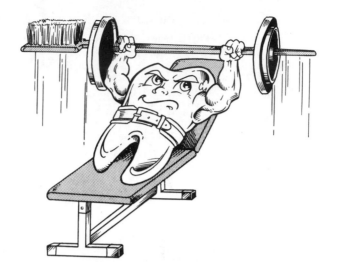

Introduction 3

How to Use This Book

Tooth Fitness is a user-friendly book—conveniently divided into three parts, with a table of contents that makes subjects easy to find, as well as a detailed index and a glossary. If you're a person who usually skips the introduction I suggest that you take a few minutes to read the rest of this one, because it contains important information that will help you use this book in the most effective way.

This book is designed to be used in conjunction with the support you'll receive from your dental team. As such, your registered dental hygienist (RDH) and dentist may want to modify my suggestions. Your mouth is one of a kind, and because they will be the ones actually looking in your mouth and evaluating your individual needs, I ask that you defer to them and follow their advice—as long as it gets results.

STEP 1: YOU WILL ACTUALLY NEED TO READ IT

I know what you're thinking: isn't there an easier way? Well, you could try sleeping on the book (maybe osmosis will occur) or talk someone into reading it to you. But when all is said and done, I think you're stuck with actually having to read it yourself. So, browse through it and look at some of Aaron's great drawings. After you get a feel for the book, you should begin your reading with Part One.

Part One ◆ Dental Disease

This section contains all you need to know about dental disease, from cause to treatment to prevention, along with everything in between. It's required reading if you sincerely want to kick the dental disease habit and get your master's degree in prevention. It lays out what you have to do for yourself—no one else can do it for you. It's a good idea to read both Parts One and Two before you have your first visit with the dentist and hygienist.

Part Two ◆ The Dental Team and You

These chapters show you how find a dentist and a hygienist, what to expect at the dental office, and how to work with the hygienist, the dentist, and the front office staff. This is must reading if you don't have a dentist but are looking for one, and worthwhile even if you have one already.

Part Three ◆ The Rest of the Story: Read It When You Need It

This section contains all kinds of important information, including some that you may need on short notice, like how to deal with an unwelcome dental emergency, and you'll want it to always be handy. This part of the book is like an insurance policy; you only have to use it once for it to pay back the cost of the book, many times over.

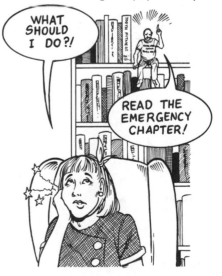

Depending on your individual oral situation, you may decide to read all of Part Three, some of it, or none of it. If your only interest is to free yourself of dental disease, Parts One and Two will take care of that. But if you really want to become a complete dental patient Part Three will be indispensable. If you have not already done so, take a look at Part Three in the table of contents. Every chapter in this section is chock-full of important information. Of course I may be a bit biased, but I think the whole section is valuable—and worth reading just for the fun of it.

Once you've finished reading Parts One and Two, and all of Part Three that you feel is necessary to read at this time, I suggest you find a good place to rest the book. It's worked hard. Put it in a spot you can remember so that you can find it when you need it. Having *Tooth Fitness* nearby will be as close as you may get to having me available in your own home.

STEP 2: TAKE IT TO THE DENTAL OFFICE

I suggest you do this for every appointment until you receive a clean bill of oral health from your RDH or dentist. I ask you to do this for a number of reasons.

First of all, it shows you care. You know you care and I know you care, but you want to make sure your dentist and hygienist know you care. Why should they think you don't care? Well, whenever you see a new dentist or hygienist, and they see fillings, decay, and gum disease, guess what they might be thinking? Try this on for size: "Obviously, this patient has seen other dentists. Someone must have talked to him at some point about prevention, but he still has dental disease. Hmmm . . . maybe he doesn't care that much about his teeth." Believe me, I know from experience that given a situation like this, these assumptions are easy to make. Thus, whatever reasons you may have had for ignoring your mouth—you never cared about it, you never had access to the preventive information, you couldn't understand the information when it was presented, you didn't follow through with your program—you don't want the dentist, or hygienist, to use your past as a gauge by which to judge you now. The best way to change their attitude is to tell your dental team that you really do care. You don't have to shout or jump up and down, but do let them know at the first opportunity that you have a new attitude toward your oral health and that you're seeking their help to *adios* this disease, forever. If you do that in a sincere and committed way, they aren't likely to draw any negative conclusions about your previous attitude. This means they'll reserve judgment until they know from their own direct experience that you've been given a real chance to take responsibility for your dental health.

When you walk into the office with this book under your arm there is a 95 percent chance that they will instantly know you do care about your mouth, without you ever saying a word. They'll recognize you as a person who is much more motivated, knowledgeable, and aware than the typical dental patient. And you'll probably be given better service and treatment. I say that because whenever patients showed me that they were serious and appreciated my help, I always directed extra energy toward their care. But never forget that the responsibility isn't all the dentist's or hygienist's. I guarantee that you won't be able to fool anyone by simply giving lip-service to caring; you will actually have to *make a firm commitment and convert that caring into action.*

There is a special section in the Appendix for questions and notes. Use it to jot down any questions you may have about your dental health, and bring your book to your dental appointment. Remember, there is no such thing as a dumb question when you're in search of knowledge, when you're trying to save your teeth, or when you're paying for the answer.

There's also a section in the Appendix where you can record the special instructions you may receive from the dentist and the

DR. TOM'S TIPS

If you feel you've tried everything and you can't obtain satisfactory answers to your questions, there are a few other things you can do. One is to ask your dental team to refer you to another dentist or dental hygienist who they feel may have answers. It could very well be that your question can be answered only by a dental specialist. You can also write to Tooth Fitness, Inc. We draw from a vast pool of information, and the chances are awfully good that we'll be able to come up with an answer. Our address is in the Appendix. We also publish a newsletter, *The Tooth Fitness Digest*, which, along with keeping you up-to-date on the latest in prevention, deals with difficult or unique dental problems. For more details on this, see the Appendix.

RDH. There's another section to record the information they'll give you about the preventive tools you'll need to accomplish your goals, along with how, when, and where to use them. All these instructions are crucial for the success of your home care program. They provide the means by which your oral hygiene program is customized to fit your individual needs. Because the stress and anxiety that may accompany you to the dental office often make it difficult to remember what you've learned there, writing it down is the best way to ensure you'll always have access to it.

There is also ample room in the Appendix for a permanent record of everything else that's important to your oral hygiene program. Such records will be valuable if you move, if your dental records are lost, or for legal matters.

I think it's a good idea to keep the copies of your *periodontal pocket charts* that your RDH will give you (you'll learn about pockets—and I don't mean the ones in your pants—soon enough) with your copy of *Tooth Fitness*. That way, as time goes by, these charts and your own notes and records will become a sort of dental diary chronicling your journey to oral health.

READ ONLY WHAT YOU NEED

Even though you may feel that you're pretty well versed about a particular subject, I suggest you read pertinent sections anyway because you just might find out something you didn't know. That missing piece could make a big difference. If you really feel confident about a certain subject, like how to find the right toothbrush, feel free to move on to another topic. However,

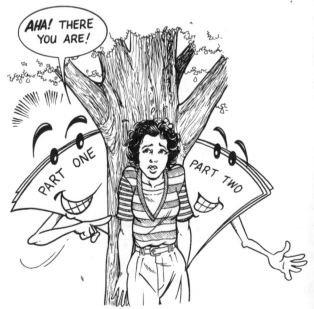

if you sincerely want this program to work for you there is no way you can escape from reading Parts One and Two.

THE PEP TALK

Maybe you thought I'd forgotten the pep talk . . . Nope. I wouldn't do that to you. However, I'll be giving you many others as we go along, so I'll make this a short one.

The book and your dental team are going to motivate and energize you and help you to make a significant change in your dental life. You'll be trading one set of habits for another—in this case, a bad set for a good set. You should understand that actually making this change takes more energy than just thinking about it. If you already have a strong wish to change, that wish will provide you with much of the energy you need to overcome the resistance of your old habits. This isn't meant to imply that there's no hope for you if you don't happen to feel motivated right now. But wait—you must be *somewhat* motivated. After all, there must be some reason you're reading this book. Is it pure chance? Fate? Trust that it was meant to be. Give your dental team and *Tooth Fitness* a chance, and see how much difference *you* can make in creating, and maintaining, a healthy mouth. I'm going to use every technique I know to stimulate your involvement, including humor and encouragement . . . Are you motivated yet? If you're not, I bet you will be by the time you're halfway through this book.

Tooth Fitness does not blame, accuse, or threaten. Neither you nor your dentist, the hygienist, your mom, or your great-great-grandfather's genes are to blame for poor dental health. The only shoulders I can find upon which to place the blame are those of ignorance. By the time you finish the book your ignorance will be a thing of the past. I might poke or prod you, and pull a leg or two, but I'll never blame you for the state of your oral health. Neither, I suspect, will your dental team. That also means that there's no room for guilt. Guilt is a waste of energy, and it only gets in the way of making positive change. Besides, if after reading *Tooth Fitness* you're still not motivated to do something for your dental health, still do not care about what happens to your mouth, you'll only be out a few bucks and you can go ahead and feel as guilty as you want then. Deal?

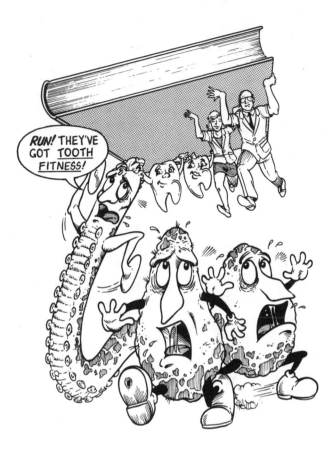

It is now time to get down to business, so read on and participate in the miracles of healing and empowerment.

One last thing: The dentist will be referred to as a male throughout the book even though, I'm glad to report, there are an increasing number of women practicing dentistry. The dental hygienist, or RDH, will be referred to as a woman. This is not intended to slight men, for there are male hygienists. However, the choice of gender reflects current statistics regarding the occupation of roles in the dental profession and is only meant to simplify your reading.

PART ONE

Dental Disease

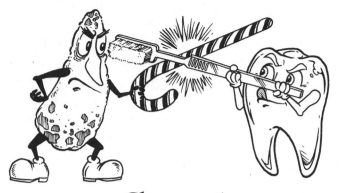

Chapter 1

Know Thy Enemy: The Truth about Tooth Decay

Dental disease is not an obscure and mysterious ailment. You didn't inherit dental disease from your mom or your grandfather. It's not something that was left behind by visiting aliens. You don't get it from kissing, and in spite of what some people believe, it certainly isn't part of a secret plot by the dental profession to stir up business.

Dental disease is not only a disease of the mouth but also a disease of the body. Any time part of your body becomes diseased, it stresses your entire body's immune system. The stress can be most harmful when the disease is a chronic one, which is the form of dental disease

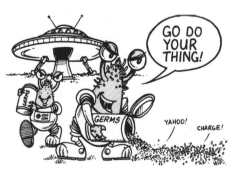

from which most patients suffer. Dental disease, especially gum disease, starts slowly, increases in severity, and then tenaciously hangs on, overloading your body's protective defenses twenty-four hours a day, for as long as you have the disease. Not only does this drain you of energy, it ends up drastically lowering your resistance to any other disease to which you may be exposed. When you look at it this way, you can no longer afford to think of dental disease as an insignificant or harmless condition that affects only your teeth.

There are many types of dental disease, but the two that will concern you the most are tooth decay and gum disease. These diseases aren't the same—not in their cause, their severity, their treatment, or their cost to you. You can have both at the same time or one without the other. Because they're so common, and the vehicles of so much pain and destruction, the focus of the first part of *Tooth Fitness* will be on their cause, treatment, and prevention.

Learning how to take care of your mouth is not difficult. Fortunately, you don't have to become a dentist or a hygienist to learn how to become an enlightened patient. But you do have to understand the basics of what you're up against in order to overcome dental disease. This chapter explains tooth decay, not because it's the most serious form of dental disease, but because it's the most familiar. Chapter 2 looks at what I consider to be your mouth's number one enemy, gum disease.

Remember the words of that famous philosopher and scholar, Anonymous: "If you don't change it, it sure as heck will stay the same." Ready? Good. So am I.

TOOTH DECAY—THE INSIDE STORY

All tooth decay, in one way or another, is related to diet. As we've become more civilized, our diet has become more refined, processed, overcooked, and overpreserved. As we've developed new processing techniques and made more of this type of food available to more people, the incidence of decay has risen proportionately. In other words, as we change our naturally balanced diet with so-called advances in food technology, without making corresponding changes in oral hygiene, we are literally creating tooth decay. Thus it really is a man-made disease, another by-product of our wild rush toward progress. Progress is a good-news/bad-news venture; while it has given us many good things, it has also made us more susceptible to dental disease.

The cause of tooth decay is pretty straightforward, and once you understand the process, it will make freeing yourself from it a heck of a lot easier. In order for decay to occur in your teeth, three things are necessary: germs, food, and teeth.

1. Germs Even though only a few types of germs (bacteria) are directly involved in tooth decay, hundreds are found in your mouth. They come in all sizes and shapes: little germs and big germs, long ones and round ones. You will have to take my word for that, because they're so small that no matter how hard you look for them, you'll never see them with the naked eye. Except for right now, that is. You may be the first to see them like this, so don't be too surprised if they look a little indignant. (If you happen to be a biologist you'll know we have taken certain liberties in characterizing and drawing germs, but as you'll see, the process we describe is accurate.)

2. Food By "food," I don't mean just any kind. The foods that are most responsible for decay are highly refined and processed carbohydrates. Once the refining is over they are known by another name, sugar. There are many kinds of sugars, but when it comes to causing decay, *sucrose* (more commonly known as white sugar) is the most destructive. (Chapter 16, "Nutrition and Your Teeth," describes the role diet plays in the health of your mouth and body. Don't miss it.)

3. Teeth You guessed it! Teeth are an indispensable part of this trio. Without them you'd never get decay, but then you would not get to eat corn on the cob either. Some teeth are harder than others and may resist decay longer, but the decay process is the same no matter how quickly or slowly it proceeds.

These three ingredients need a nice, cozy place to get together, and your mouth fills this requirement to a T. But in order for the germs to really do a number on your teeth, they also need as much freedom from the brush, the floss, the water irrigation device, your hygienist, and the dentist as they can get. I'm not pointing any fingers, but don't you think you might have been helping them out (unconsciously, I'm sure) by providing them with the environment they so dearly love? If you have been giving them free rein you're not alone. In most of us (except the over 13 million people with no teeth), there exists the potential for tooth decay.

Let's get some background material on the germs that have helped create all of this oral havoc.

Germ Facts

Here are some little-known facts about those little buggers that love boring holes into your precious choppers.

1. Size As I've said, these characters are small—even smaller than small. Just how small are they? Well, small enough that millions of them can fit onto an area the size of this dot (.). By the way, did you know that there are more germs in a diseased mouth than there are stars in our Milky Way galaxy?

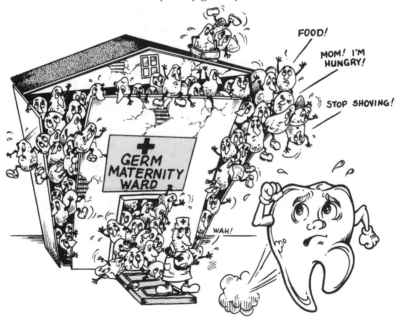

2. Sexuality Sexually, germs are truly amazing. Their birthrate is simply outrageous. Given the proper conditions, which most of us give them regularly, one germ can produce millions of offspring in a few hours. The concept of family planning has escaped them entirely.

3. Life-style Unlike humans, the germs that cause tooth decay don't need oxygen to survive. This is important in the decay

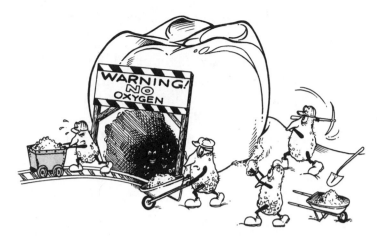

process because, even after they have tunneled their way into your tooth's enamel, where there's no air supply, they continue to eat, eliminate, reproduce, and tunnel some more. They also love it when they are left under fillings, can sneak in under a flaw in a filling, or are protected by the plaque and calculus that shield them from the brush and decay-fighting saliva.

4. Will to live   Germs are tenacious characters. If it were not for the fact that they can cause so much damage to your teeth and gums, I'd admire such tenacity. As a group they have survived everything human beings have tried to do to get rid of them and have come out unscathed. It's not as if they're mean or inherently evil. Like us, they're just trying to survive. In a healthy mouth they are kept in balance and cause no dental problems. We're the ones who have turned them into monsters by continuing to feed their insatiable appetites. These microscopic little guys were here before we were, and I think there's a good chance they may still be here long after we're gone.

5. Habits   In my opinion, germs are addicts. They're not addicted to cigarettes, alcohol, heroin, or caffeine, but they do love sucrose. Their sugar addiction is so bad that if you leave foods containing sugar in your mouth (heaven forbid) they would go on eating and eating and eating and eating, twenty-four hours a day. The waste that these germs eliminate as a by-product of digestion, also twenty-four hours a day, is very acidic—a biological and chemical fact that does not bode well for your teeth. The important thing is to keep these germs from congregating in one place for any length of time. You can control their population by controlling what you feed them and by keeping your teeth clean.

6. *Diet* Germs don't need a lot of food to do well in their world. In fact, they need only microscopic amounts to survive and multiply like lemmings. The food that you might leave in your mouth doesn't seem like it would support any living body, but you can bet your car's pink slip it can support about 10 zillion germ bodies. And once they penetrate your tooth's *enamel* (the outermost protective layer) and get into the *dentin* (the tooth structure found under the enamel), they no longer need an outside source of food. Why? Because now they have a handy source of living food—your dentin—and it is unlimited. When you realize how much dentin there is in each tooth and how microscopic the germs are, it's easy to see that they have enough food to live on for billions and billions of their lifetimes. And the more germs there are, the more of your enamel they destroy and the more dentin they eat. This may sound like morbid humor, but how does it feel to know a part of your body is slowly being eaten alive by these little carnivores?

These germ characteristics play a very important role in the decay process. Before we learn how that process works, let's take a quick look at a decay-free environment. (In case you're wondering, fluoridated teeth are an exception to the rule. See Chapter 18 for a discussion of fluoride's effect on tooth decay and gum disease.)

A Decay-Free Mouth

A decay-free mouth requires the following:

☐ Freedom from germ food (food containing sucrose)

☐ A stabilized germ population, controlled by your mouth's defenses and your oral hygiene program

☐ A normal saliva flow, which protects the teeth by neutralizing the harmful acids that germs eliminate after dining on the free meals you provide

ACID AND THE BEGINNING OF DECAY

The only time germs can cause a healthy tooth to become decayed is when you don't keep your mouth free of germ food. If you don't keep your mouth clean you give germs the opportunity to vastly and rapidly increase their population. The result is that all the little acid-producing germs combine to create one big decay-producing factory.

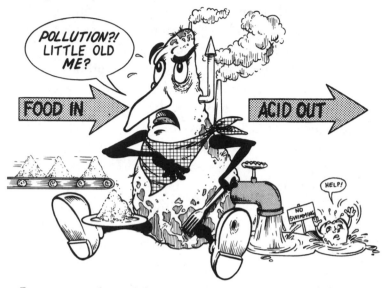

Once a member of the germ gang has eaten and digested the sugar that you left for them, he does the same thing you eventually do: he eliminates his waste products. This elimination process is as natural a function for germs as it is for us, except germs do it all day and all night long. This acid waste, if undiluted and left in contact with the tooth, is actually powerful enough to dissolve your tooth's enamel, which is the hardest substance in your body. If you multiply one germ's acid output by billions of his buddies, you end up with more acid than your saliva can possibly neutralize. When that happens, the decay process begins.

The key to preventing the decay process is this: the three items that combine to cause decay—germs, germ food, and teeth—must not be allowed to be present at the same time. Obviously, we can't eliminate all the germs, and I doubt if anyone would be in favor of eliminating the teeth. Let's see . . . that leaves germ food! We're in luck, because germ food can be eliminated.

Sucrose: A Germ's Favorite Food

Germs can't order out—their menu is our menu. But they do have their preferences, and their small size limits what they can eat to very small things. However, because germs can only eat very small things, their choice is pretty much restricted to refined sugars, the smallest and simplest of the carbohydrates. Carbohydrates are a class of energy-producing foods. Some are complex, like starches and cellulose, and some are simple, like sucrose (white sugar). Most of the carbohydrates found in natural foods are too large and too complex to be broken down into sucrose either by chewing or by the enzymes found in your mouth. So complex carbohydrates don't make good germ food. But simple carbohydrates—especially refined sugars—are another story. Just think what would happen to your teeth if germs could digest any kind of food that gets left in your mouth. Your teeth wouldn't have a prayer of surviving. (It shouldn't take too much imagination to visualize a world in which we all buy dentures in the supermarket.)

The refining of foods, in the simplest terms, is a process by which the original, whole, and natural food is broken down into many smaller parts. This alteration is most dramatically illustrated by the refining process that creates white sugar. Most plants naturally contain small amounts of sucrose, as well as other simple sugars, but the plant must undergo a refining process for the sucrose to be extracted. The sugar beet and sugarcane are the two most commonly used plants from which white sugar is extracted. I flipped a coin to see which to use to demonstrate the refining process, and the sugar beet won.

In its natural state, the sugar beet is a pretty stout-looking character. No self-respecting germ would ever take him on. But when that hardy character is refined, the picture changes drastically. The refining process reduces poor Mr. Beet down to one of the smallest sizes to which a carbohydrate can be reduced and still be

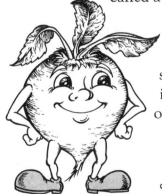

called a food—if white sugar can ever be called a food. (In my opinion, and that of many others, it should be classified as a drug, and an addictive one at that.) When simple white sugar is left in the mouth, even in small quantities, it provides the trillions of starving germs with enough food to allow them to commit the hideous crime of tooth decay.

Bear in mind that any processed food containing sucrose can

cause the same result as plain old white sugar. And be wary of so-called natural foods, because even they can contain sugar. So be sure to read the label. There are manufacturers who claim white sugar is natural just because it comes from a natural source and don't hesitate to use it in their "natural" products.

It's really pretty simple: the more sugar a food contains, the faster it will cause tooth decay.

A Germ's Least Favorite Foods

Even after a good chewing, most of the carbohydrates in natural (unrefined and unprocessed) food are still so much larger than the average germ that germs can't possibly digest them. The amount of accessible sugars, including sucrose, released from chewing most fruits, vegetables, and grains is so small that it's not a significant factor in the normal decay process. And although the enzymes found in saliva do initiate the breakdown of complex carbohydrates and prepare them for complete digestion in the intestines, they can't break them down into sucrose in the mouth.

But no enzymes are needed to reduce sucrose to the size germs like. These sugar molecules are already bite-size, and the germs can begin feasting on them immediately upon contact.

I've given you a general idea of the sugar-refining process and why white sugar is the real villain (see Chapter 16 for more detail), and now it's time to graphically explain how all this ties together.

The Decay Experiments

In the interest of scientific knowledge (though certainly not in the interest of the animals tested), some very original experiments were performed to show the relationship between natural foods, refined foods, germs, and tooth decay. The following experiments demonstrate what I call the "triad theory" of tooth decay. In the simplest of terms, if you want tooth decay, just invite your teeth, decay-causing food, and germs to the same party. If you don't, leave one of them off the guest list.

Group A experiment In part 1 of the experiment, the mouths and the surrounding environment of a group of laboratory animals were sterilized in order to remove all the germs. These animals were then fed a diet consisting solely of white sugar. This diet was contin-

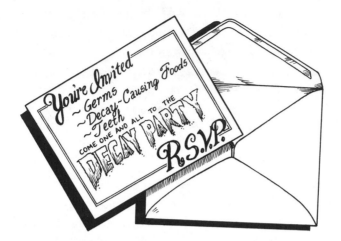

ued for a set period of time. At the end of that period they were examined and the researchers found no decay. There is, of course, a very good reason for this, and I know that you've figured it out. Yep, one of the three requirements for decay had been removed—the germs. Which means no one was at the dinner table to eat and digest the decay-causing sucrose that was abundantly available. Therefore, no acid was produced and there was no decay.

In the second part of the experiment, large quantities of germs were introduced to the same animals who participated in part 1. They were then fed the same amount of sugar, but this time through a tube connected to their stomachs. The idea here was to keep any food from touching the teeth and mingling with the germs now in their mouths. The researchers wanted to see if large numbers of decay-causing germs kept in constant contact with teeth but deprived of refined foods could cause decay. Again, lo and behold, no decay was found in any of the animals. Why? Again, one of the trio was missing; this time it was refined food. The experiment conclusively demonstrated that even with a vast increase in the germ population, germs can't cause decay on their own. They must eat sugar to cause tooth decay.

Part 3 of the experiment, the ultimate test, was soon carried out. The same, still decay-free, animals that were used in the first two parts were used again. This time both sucrose and decay-causing germs were introduced *at the same time.* This third phase lasted the same amount of time as the previous two phases—apples for apples. The results showed that the same teeth that seemed to be decay-proof were now rapidly decaying. This was to be expected. For the first time in the experiment, all three of the trio were found together at the same time—germs, teeth, and sucrose.

In part 4 of the experiment, the same animals were used, and all of the animals' teeth were extracted. (I personally do not think this was necessary to prove the point, but researchers are sticklers for detail.) The animals were fed the same decay-causing diet and were pumped full of decay-causing germs. The test lasted the same amount of time as the previous three. The difference was that the animals had no teeth. In its own inhumane way, this test also proved the triad theory: when you remove one of the three ingredients, decay can't take place.

This should, once and for all, make it perfectly clear that there is truly a direct cause-and-effect relationship between diet, germs, and tooth decay. You can now forget every other theory you have ever heard about the cause of tooth decay.

EXPERIMENT A

Part	Teeth	Type of Food	Germs	Results
1	Yes	Sucrose	None	NO DECAY
2	Yes	None	Present	NO DECAY
3	Yes	Sucrose	Present	DECAY
4	No	Sucrose	Present	NO DECAY

Group B experiment The researchers didn't stop with one experiment. They wanted to find out what would happen if the animals were allowed to consume a natural diet. I salute them for that.

In the first part of experiment B, the researchers used the same kind of animals that took part in experiment A. Again the germs were eliminated from their mouths, but in this experiment, their diet consisted of the food found in their natural environment. See if you can come up with the answer before you read it. Right: no decay. Reason? Right again: one part of the trio didn't show up for the party—the germ crowd.

In the second part of this experiment, the animals were again fed through a tube, and the germs were reinstated in abundance. Results? Again, no decay. Reason? One of the three amigos was missing. (This story might be getting a little predictable, but don't get too complacent, there's an interesting twist to it.)

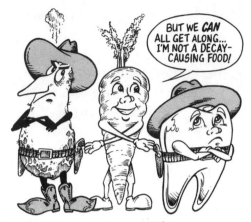

In part 3, the natural food was left for the germs to eat, the teeth were left in place, and zillions upon zillions of bacteria were pumped back into the mouth. Results? No decay. But wait just a minute. That seems to shoot down the triad theory because in this experiment all three ingredients were found together, yet no decay occurred. Hmmm? When all three were combined in experiment A, the teeth decayed like wildfire. Well, the theory still holds true; we simply need to distinguish between decay-causing food and natural, healthy food.

There was one more part of experiment B . . . the coup de grace. In part 4, all the animals in group B, still decay-free, had their natural diet replaced by the same refined diet that was fed to the group A animals. Everything else remained the same. Result? Their teeth decayed. Reason? The refined-food-loving bacteria got their diet of choice and did what they'll do every time those conditions exist—rot the teeth.

EXPERIMENT B

Part	Teeth	Type of Food	Germs	Results
1	Yes	Natural	None	NO DECAY
2	No	None	Yes	NO DECAY
3	Yes	Natural	Yes	NO DECAY
4	Yes	Sucrose	Yes	DECAY

These experiments demonstrate two important ideas that are necessary for you to understand your battle against tooth decay:

1. How decay happens

2. The role refined foods play in the decay process

As long as you don't eat foods containing white sugar, or if you remove the remains of these foods from your mouth *immediately* after eating, *you will never get tooth decay again.*

WHEN ACID MEETS DENTIN

Okay, let's get back to what happens when the acid produced by germs hits your teeth. In order for the acid to etch its way through the enamel (which, you'll remember, is the hardest substance in the body), it has to be concentrated, in constant contact with the tooth, and protected from both saliva and the toothbrush. Plaque, which adheres to the teeth, is a mixture of germs, food particles, and dead and living cells—a perfect medium that allows all three conditions to exist. (Plaque is discussed in detail in Chapter 2.) The decay-causing germs congregate in the plaque, where the acids they produce become concentrated and are protected. So although plaque itself doesn't directly *cause* decay, it certainly promotes it.

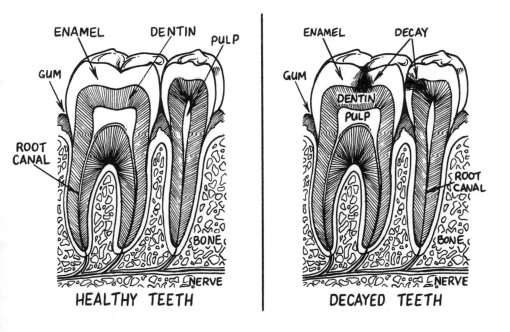

HEALTHY TEETH   DECAYED TEETH

And now what? Well, when those little germs have used their acids to etch a tunnel through the enamel and have reached the dentin, you are past the point of being able to prevent further damage with home care alone. Now the damage will have to be repaired by the dentist. Part of the tooth's dentin is organic and not nearly as hard as the inorganic enamel. Not only can the acid dissolve dentin more easily and faster than enamel, but about 30 percent of the dentin exists in a form that can be eaten by the germs. This means that even if you were to hone your oral hygiene skills to perfection and always remove every particle of food from your mouth immediately after eating, you would still be unable to stop the destruction from taking place under fillings or in the tunnels bored by acid. The initial tunnel is so small that no brush can gain access to it; even your decay-fighting saliva cannot reach into this microscopic tunnel. Therefore the destruction will continue unabated. If you interviewed a germ and asked him what would be an ideal situation in which to live happily ever after, the one I just described would be the one he would choose.

As you have no way of seeing or feeling when the germs have reached the dentin, you should now be better able to appreciate the value of a dental examination, including a full-mouth series of X rays. Only an X ray will reveal the extent of the decay. Unless X rays are used to detect decay, you won't know what's happening until the pain comes. And if that has ever happened to you, you know what a miserable experience it can be.

SUSCEPTIBLE AREAS

There are many parts of the tooth that are difficult to keep clean and thus are vulnerable to decay, but the two prime locations are the *occlusal grooves* and the *contact points*.

Grooves

Grooves (or *fissures*, as they are called by the pros) are found on the tops, or occlusal (grinding) surfaces, of the molars and bicuspids. If you look at the cusps of teeth as hills, the grooves are the canyons that form between them. Grooves are formed as the tooth develops. Unfortunately, the enamel at the bottom of these grooves is usually so thin that it doesn't take the acid long to penetrate it and reach the dentin. The problem is made worse by the fact that toothbrush bristles are too thick to fit into the grooves. This makes these grooves terrific plaque traps, and once plaque is formed in them, no amount of brushing or fluoride treatments will be able to keep them from decaying.

The grooves on the occlusal surfaces of the back teeth, especially in the thin, soft enamel of baby teeth, are especially vulner-

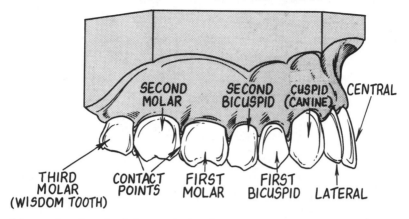

NAMES OF THE TEETH

SECOND MOLAR · SECOND BICUSPID · CUSPID (CANINE) · CENTRAL

THIRD MOLAR (WISDOM TOOTH) · CONTACT POINTS · FIRST MOLAR · FIRST BICUSPID · LATERAL

able to this kind of decay. (Nearly 60 percent of all the cavities in children are found in the fissures of their back teeth, both baby and permanent.) In these cases they should be filled or cleaned out and preventively treated with sealants. However, not all grooves will need to be filled. A simple check by the dentist, with the aid of his trusty *explorer* (a thin, curved, metal pick), will tell you which ones will need treatment.

Contact Points

The next most vulnerable area is the contact point, the area where two teeth touch. This area is susceptible to decay because when food is forced between the teeth it often gets stuck there. Once this happens, germs congregate, plaque forms, and decay soon follows. Contact points are extremely vulnerable because the bristles of the toothbrush cannot reach them. Dental floss is the most effective preventive measure.

Other Susceptible Areas

Pits and defects Pits and defects can be found anywhere on a tooth but are most often found on the backs of the cuspids, on the cusps, and on the backs of the front teeth (centrals and laterals). These irregularities in the enamel result from improper formation while the tooth is developing. They are food and plaque traps, and like grooves, most can't be kept clean. As with grooves, not all will develop decay, but they all should be checked, then filled or smoothed out to prevent food and plaque from accumulating.

Roots If bone loss and the inevitable gum recession have taken place, the exposed roots become extremely susceptible to decay. They're not covered by protective enamel, and the food and plaque now have access to the spaces that once were filled by bone and gums. These areas are difficult to fill and to keep clean—brushing alone won't be sufficient here. Root decay is a very serious problem for people over sixty.

Margins A *margin* is the term dentists use to describe the seam where the tooth and the filling meet. Margins are very vulnerable to decay because even the best-fitting filling, when viewed microscopically, is rough, has gaps and defects, and is an ideal hang-out for food, germs, and plaque.

Underneath fillings The tooth structure underneath fillings is another area where decay can recur, but only if all the decay was not removed when the tooth was prepared for the filling. Sometimes, but not always, X rays will show if there's decay under a filling. This depends on the type of filling. For example, if a tooth has a full crown, the X rays can't penetrate the crown's metal. Learning how to pick the best and most conscientious dentist is the best way to prevent this type of decay.

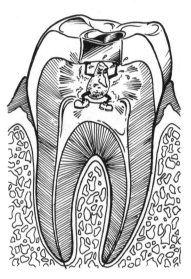

Smooth Surfaces

The smooth surfaces of a tooth, except around the gum line and the contacts, are normally not susceptible to decay. Because of the action of the tongue, the lips, and the cheeks, as well as the cleansing action of food and saliva, these areas are generally kept free of plaque and the germs that hang out in it.

SOMETHING TO THINK ABOUT

As destructive as tooth decay can be, most damaged teeth can be repaired—if you can afford it, that is. It's true that fluoridation has reduced the incidence of decay in our society. But everything is relative. When you consider the fact that the average six-year-old has one decayed, missing, or filled tooth, and that the same child will have twenty-two decayed, missing, or filled teeth by the time he's in his sixties, you will probably agree with me that decay is still a serious problem.

Teeth are not inanimate objects that you can buy or rent. They're as much a part of your body as your eyes, ears, hands, and heart. When you view them in that way it should motivate you to want to take care of them. But even if you don't get decay, or have had all the susceptible areas filled, you're not yet out of the woods— because the real killer of teeth is gum disease.

You may think gum disease is not your problem, and you might be right. But then again, you might be wrong. Gum disease is now the most prevalent form of dental disease for everyone over thirty. (By the way, how old are you now?) Maybe you're not too concerned about gum disease, but I've a feeling that those people over sixty who don't have a single tooth left (45 percent), or who have lost half their teeth (14 percent), also didn't think gum disease would be a problem. Now that I have you thinking about it, let's find out more about this nasty disease.

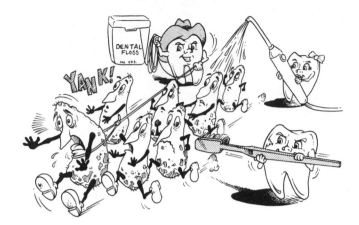

Chapter 2

Gum Disease

Gum disease is less commonly known as *periodontal disease*. Although the term *gum disease* is a familiar one and easy to remember, it is not an altogether accurate term, and it doesn't convey the seriousness of the disease. (In this book, I use the two terms interchangeably.) Learning the proper terminology for the various forms of dental disease will make it easier for you to communicate with your hygienist and dentist, because they may use "in-house" terminology to explain your condition to you. Whatever words they use, make sure you understand the concepts and issues that apply to your case.

The dental community acknowledges two main stages of periodontal (meaning "around the tooth") disease. The first is a disease of the gums, or *gingivae*, called *gingivitis*. The second is called *periodontitis*, which is a disease of the ligament and bone that hold your teeth in your jaws. Although these two forms of periodontal disease are the most serious forms of dental disease, they've never been given enough recognition by the public for the destruction they can cause. Tooth decay wounds, but the real killer of teeth is periodontal disease. If we had a criminal penal code for classifying dental disease, decay would be considered a misdemeanor and periodontal disease would be a felony. Most tooth decay can be repaired, but once advanced gum disease destroys the bone that supports the teeth in your jaws, those teeth will be lost forever. When that happens, even King Midas wouldn't have enough money to save them.

It's one thing to think you might have a little gum problem; it's another thing entirely to realize that this disease is actually destroying the tissues, ligaments, and bones of your body. If you knew that the tissues, ligaments, and bones of your arm, for example, were slowly being destroyed, and would eventually be lost because of infection, you'd be very concerned, to say the least, and you would do whatever you could to treat it. Am I right? Well, the tissues, ligaments, and bones in your mouth are every bit as much a part of your body as those of your arm. Ponder that for a few moments.

THE CAUSE OF PERIODONTAL DISEASE

You have probably read, or been told, that the cause of periodontal disease is anything from a poor diet, germs, bad genes, plaque, or calculus (tartar) to kissing too much or not enough. There may be a bit of truth to each of these, but when you get right down to it, the primary cause of periodontal disease is *poor oral hygiene*. Whether you have this disease because you didn't know how to prevent it, or you just didn't care, the results are the same. As they say, ignorance is no excuse in the eyes of the law.

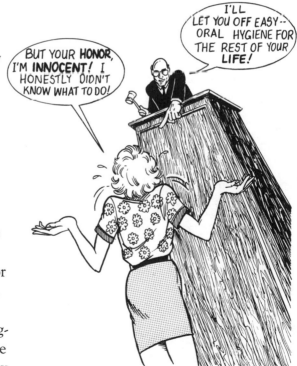

Although poor oral hygiene is the main cause of periodontal disease, there are other significant factors that affect its onset, extent, and severity: the germ population of your mouth, your general health, genetics, your bite, your age, diet, your life-style (smoking, drinking, etc.), stress, drug side effects, and your relationship with your hygienist and dentist.

CLASSIFYING GUM DISEASE: GINGIVITIS AND PERIODONTITIS

Periodontal disease is complicated by the fact that different types of disease can exist in different areas of your mouth at the same time. The severity of gingivitis and periodontitis can vary from one tooth to another and even from one part of a tooth to another, meaning different stages of disease can occur simultaneously around the the same tooth. With periodontal disease there is no clear-cut visual way for you to tell exactly when irritation and inflammation turn into gingivitis or when gingivitis ends and periodontitis begins.

DR. TOM'S TIPS

Most forms of gum disease progress slowly, and there's no way for you to accurately determine how severe it is without a detailed examination by the hygienist or dentist.

Stage 1 Periodontal Disease: Gingivitis

Gingivitis is the most common form of periodontal disease. In simple terms, it is an inflammation of the gum tissue. Uncared for, the inflammation turns into more serious forms of infection and eventually evolves into periodontitis. The most common way to classify gingivitis is by cause and severity. Generally, it's enough to know that it has three phases, and if, for example, you are in the third phase you have the most serious form. Your hygienist will guide you in determining what caused your gingivitis and what phase it is in, but it's important for you to be familiar with the most common types.

Simple gingivitis Over 90 percent of all Americans have had, have now, or will have this form of gum disease. It can occur around one, or all, of your teeth. The first sign is a reddish, shiny band that is seen at the point where the gums meet the teeth. In the early stages of the disease the gums may not bleed, but they will as the disease progresses. This condition can arise in as little as a week if the teeth and gums aren't cared for. If caught soon enough you can treat it yourself. With the right attention, and depending on how serious it is, it should heal in one to three weeks. If you can't reverse this process in that amount of time you'll need the help of the hygienist.

Chronic gingivitis At this stage, the disease is no longer simple. Chronic gingivitis is like an old tree with widespread roots that are entrenched and difficult to remove. This is a very common form of periodontal disease in patients who brush enough to keep the disease from moving rapidly but not enough to stop it. The rate this disease progresses will be a direct reflection of the amount of time you spend taking care of teeth, your diet, how fast you form plaque, and how efficiently the plaque was removed. Generally, the areas of the mouth that receive the least attention are the ones that are the most affected. This stage of the disease may not be painful, but there is inflammation and infection, and bleeding will take place occasionally. It's important to note that the degree of bleeding isn't always an indication of the severity of periodontal disease.

Acute gingivitis Common names for this type of gingivitis are Vincent's infection, trench mouth, and ANUG, acute necrotizing ulcerative gingivostomatatitis. If these don't scare you, nothing will. Acute gingivitis can appear suddenly and is very painful, but it usually responds well to proper treatment at the dental office. Some of the most common symptoms are fever, swollen lymph nodes, and malaise (tiredness). Its visual signs are angry, red, and swollen gums; craterlike depressions at the edges of the gums between the teeth; and gray-colored skin around the edges of the infection. The infected area will be painful when touched by anything: your finger, food, or the toothbrush. Because brushing at this stage is painful, the tendency is to cut down on the already insufficient oral care, and this only makes the condition worse. The infected area bleeds easily and is accompanied by a nasty smell.

This is the most serious form of gingivitis. It can involve one or more teeth, and it can rapidly expand to the ligament and bone if not treated. As in most forms of dental disease, the initiating cause is poor oral hygiene and the resultant plaque buildup. Many dental professionals, including myself, believe that lowered resistance, poor nutrition, and stress (possibly from other diseases) share the blame in the cause and persistence of acute gingivitis. The milder forms of gingivitis can be likened to smoldering coals just waiting to be fanned into an acute gingivitis flame. Lowered resistance, poor nutrition, and stress are the fan.

Stage 2 Periodontal Disease: Periodontitis

Periodontitis is an ominous and frightening word. It represents an ominous and frightening disease. If you have this type of periodontal disease, you are at the stage where the infection has broken through the first line of defense, the gums, and has begun to attack the ligaments and bone supporting the teeth. This is the stage where bone loss occurs, causing the *pocket (sulcus)*, the space between the gum and the tooth, to deepen. Periodontitis, like gingivitis, occurs in different forms and can involve parts of, or all of, one tooth or many teeth at the same time. Like any disease of your body, it can be treated—if it's detected in its early stages. However, if it isn't treated *you will eventually lose your teeth.*

You can certainly obtain enough information from Chapter 3, "Oral Self-Examination," to get a pretty good idea if you have the disease and which stage it's in. But any final diagnosis will be up to your dentist or the periodontist. With the right knowledge, diligent home care, hygiene therapy, and guidance from your hygienist, you'll be able to cure periodontitis, if it hasn't progressed too far.

Simple periodontitis Although simple periodontitis can be found in teenagers, it is seen more often in people over thirty, and the most serious cases are found in people over fifty. But it is definitely not limited to any age group.

This disease is characterized by chronic gum inflammation, bone loss, and a deepening of the gum pocket that range from a little to a lot. In the advanced stages tooth movement will occur. The speed at which it advances is directly related to how well you take care of your gums, both the outsides and the pockets. Simple periodontitis doesn't always involve pain, but it's usually associated with some, or all, of the following symptoms:

☐ Sensitivity to heat and cold, sugar, acidic foods, and possibly brushing. Sensitivity develops when you've had bone loss, because bone loss exposes the microscopic *tubules* in the dentin. These tubules run like pipes from the outside of the dentin into the pulp of the tooth, which contains the tooth's nerves and blood vessels (see illustrations, pages 46 and 47). When the tubules are exposed to acid, germs, air, and temperature changes, these irritants cause a pain response in the pulp.

☐ Acute and sudden pain or throbbing that is made worse by tapping on the affected tooth. This symptom points to more extensive bone loss and may also be associated with a deep abscess of the gum pocket or an infected nerve.

☐ Constant or periodic bleeding.

☐ A dull, deep, almost painlike sensation that feels as if something is putting intense pressure on the root of the tooth. Most often this is the result of food or other substances that have been jammed into the gum pocket. It is often associated with a bad contact between two teeth that allows food to be forced into the pocket. This feeling worsens the longer the irritant is left there.

☐ Toothache. Any rapidly moving decay can cause acute pain, but the toothache associated with periodontitis is usually of the throbbing variety. It's an indication that decay has started in the root and has begun to irritate the tooth's main nerve. Root decay is the only kind of decay associated with periodontitis.

Complex periodontitis The primary factors associated with complex periodontitis are the same as those found in the simple variety. However, they are complicated by the stress and trauma resulting from forces exerted on the teeth and bone. Any abnormal and long-term pressure that is placed on the bone by chewing improperly, clenching, or grinding can cause the bone to recede. Therefore, tooth movement is often seen at an early stage in complex periodontitis—earlier than in the simple form. Increased and irregular pressure is being placed on the teeth and bone because the bone is being attacked both by germs and by occlusal stress. Complex periodontitis usually progresses at a more rapid rate than the simple form.

Dentists often find that a bite problem is also associated with advanced bone loss. This is a lot like the chicken and the egg: which came first? In essence, an existing bad bite will make the existing periodontitis worse, and periodontitis will then make the bite problem worse. In other words, when you combine periodontitis and a severe bite problem, the destructive processes are accelerated.

Juvenile periodontitis   In most cases, juvenile periodontitis is found in children and young adults with other diseases, such as Down's syndrome or Papillon-Lefevre syndrome. It is believed that these diseases are not necessarily the cause of periodontitis, but contribute to it by lowering resistance and causing nutritional deficiencies that interfere with the development of bone and surrounding tissues. Juvenile periodontitis is classified according to the location of the most severe infections, that is, whether it's found around all the teeth or only involve specific teeth, usually the molars and front teeth.

Diseases caused by atrophy and by disuse   Periodontal disease can be caused by atrophy and disuse, and both conditions may exist without any active plaque involvement or any active infection.

Disease caused by atrophy is usually found in older people and is generally the result of a long time of wear and tear on the teeth and on the underlying bone that supports them. Bone loss and the resulting gum recession can occur without the presence of infection.

In periodontal disease caused by disuse, the ligament surrounding the tooth is the area most affected. Teeth are designed to chew, and when they don't, or when they don't chew normally, they become more susceptible to disease. Over time, the ligament gets

DR. TOM'S TIPS

Periodontitis is nothing to be sneezed at. It is a major threat to your health and well-being. If you have periodontitis your mouth is in serious trouble, and you must be willing to do whatever it takes to correct this problem. You must accept that once your gingivitis turns into periodontitis, it *cannot* be treated and cured with home treatment alone.

thinner and is severely weakened. This is the result of chewing improperly, eating food that is too soft, or having a misaligned bite that prevents teeth from actively participating in the chewing process. If they were now suddenly asked to do a lot of work, the affected ligaments could become tender and sore.

THE STORY OF PERIODONTAL DISEASE

To most people, their mouth is a mystery land. They've never examined their own mouth, they don't know what a healthy mouth looks like, and they have little or no idea of how gum disease begins and ends. In this section I describe how your mouth can go from a state of health to a state of toothless misery, a process that few people know about. You will follow a tooth on its journey from a healthy mouth to a jar sitting in the oral surgeon's office. Keep in mind that there are literally thousands of jars in thousands of dental offices that contain millions of teeth—teeth that, with a little care and attention, could have stayed in their owners' mouths. Though the disease can last a lifetime, the story of how it evolves is a short one.

The Cast of Characters

In order for gum disease to occur all the following characters must be on stage with you at the same time: teeth, ligaments and pockets, gums, germs, bone, plaque, calculus, food, and saliva. As in the case of tooth decay, if the participants are left on their own, in the absence of oral hygiene, you will certainly contract this disease.

Teeth   In the ideal mouth—a mouth that has never experienced any form of dental disease—each tooth has a crown; one, two, or three roots; and pulp. The *crown* (the part of the tooth above the gum line) is covered by enamel, and the *root* (which is below the gum line) is covered with *cementum*, a type of calcified tissue that is about as thick as a human hair and is softer than both enamel and dentin. (I discussed enamel and dentin in Chapter 1.) The crown and the root meet at what is called the *cemento-enamel junction* (CEJ).

The *pulp*, which contains blood vessels and nerves, leads into the *root canal*, which in turn connects to the nerves and blood vessels of the jawbone.

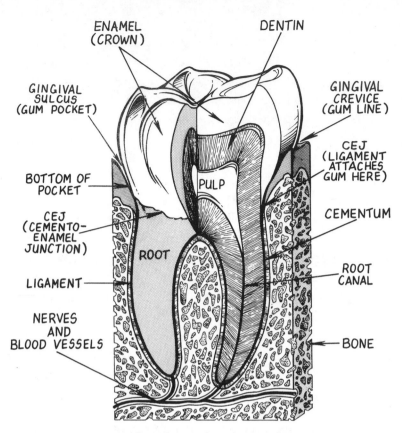

ENAMEL
(CROWN)

DENTIN

GINGIVAL
SULCUS
(GUM POCKET)

GINGIVAL
CREVICE
(GUM LINE)

CEJ
(LIGAMENT
ATTACHES
GUM HERE)

BOTTOM OF
POCKET

PULP

CEJ
(CEMENTO-
ENAMEL
JUNCTION)

CEMENTUM

ROOT

ROOT
CANAL

LIGAMENT

NERVES
AND
BLOOD VESSELS

BONE

THE ANATOMY OF A HEALTHY TOOTH

Ligaments and pockets   The *periodontal ligament* averages about one-fifth of a millimeter in width and completely surrounds the root of the tooth, filling the space between the root and the bone. It attaches the root to the bone. It has a blood and nerve supply and also serves to act as a shock absorber—helping to protect the bone from the forces exerted while chewing. Without it your teeth would fall out.

In a healthy mouth, one that has never had gum disease, the ligament and the gum join at the cemento-enamel junction. Here's where the ligament attaches the gum to the tooth, forming the bottom of the gingival sulcus, or gum pocket. The pocket, just like the pocket of your shirt, has two sides (the tooth and the gum) and a narrow bottom (where the gum and the ligament meet the tooth).

Gums   The gingiva, or gum, is really a type of specialized skin, much like the skin that covers your hands. It covers and protects the bone that surrounds the teeth. Before your baby teeth erupted,

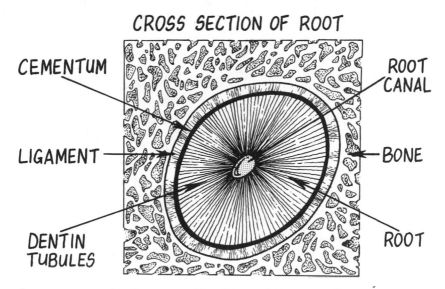

CROSS SECTION OF ROOT

CEMENTUM

ROOT CANAL

LIGAMENT

BONE

DENTIN TUBULES

ROOT

the gums completely covered both jaws. Nature, in her infinite wisdom, allowed the teeth to penetrate the gums and devised a way for the gums to stay attached to the teeth after they erupted.

As long as the gums remain free from disease, the ligament keeps it attached to the root. Healthy gums hold tightly to the tooth, closing the pocket, so to speak, and helping to prevent food and plaque from reaching the ligament, the roots, and the extremely vulnerable underlying bone.

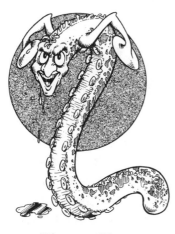

Germs As you now know, your mouth contains hundreds of types of germs. Some germs are more active in the gum disease process, but in general, the degree and seriousness of gum disease are directly proportional to the total germ population. Even in a healthy mouth, a small drop of saliva can easily contain 50 to 100 million germs, but the same amount of saliva from a diseased mouth can contain *billions* of the little monsters.

Plaque Plaque is an accumulation of germs (both dead and alive), saliva, food substances (mostly carbohydrates and proteins), dead skin cells, and the germ-fighting cells that have been released by the body to fight the bad guys. Initially it forms a sticky, nearly invisible layer that attaches to the tooth but not the gums. As it continues to grow it takes on a whitish-gray color.

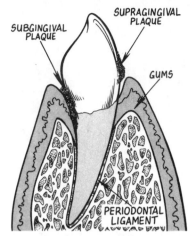

There are two kinds of plaque. They are distinguished by where they are found and their composition. The first type, *supragingival plaque*, is found above the gum line, usually on the lower third of the tooth (or upper third for top teeth), with most of the deposits found in or close to the *gingival crevice*. The second type of plaque formation is called *subgingival plaque* and is found in the gum pocket.

The main difference between the two types of plaque is that the subgingival plaque contains many more kinds of bacteria than does the supra plaque. This is because the bacteria in the pocket are protected from most of the cleansing done by the tongue, the saliva, and the toothbrush. Thus, the pocket supports more germs in general, and more of the nastier ones in particular. This, along with the fact that it is much more difficult to keep the pocket clean and healthy than it is to keep the gums around the outside of the teeth clean and healthy, makes subgingival plaque the more serious of the two. If you didn't have a germ in your mouth you would not get the infectious forms of periodontal disease. Likewise, if you never formed plaque you wouldn't get them, either.

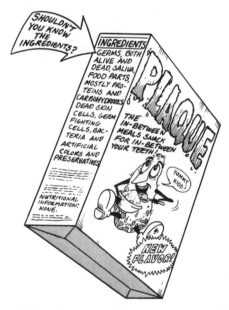

Calculus This is what plaque is called after mineral deposits have caused it to become calcified. Calculus (also called *tartar*) is composed mainly of inorganic compounds, mostly calcium phosphate, with traces of other mineral compounds. The rest of it is organic material: skin cells, dead germs, germ-fighting cells, various carbohydrates, protein, and a tiny bit of fat.

The easiest way to visualize how plaque turns into calculus is to think of a coral reef. Originally, coral is soft and is composed of living organisms. Then, because it stays in one place too long, minerals accumulate and it calcifies. Calculus is just oral coral. Plaque not only creates the matrix from which calculus starts, but also, once calculus forms, collects on top of the calculus after it has hardened. This ongoing process is like building that coral reef. First you have plaque; it hardens to form calculus; then more plaque forms on top of the calculus and hardens to form more calculus; and so on. The rate of calculus formation depends on your diet, your saliva, and your oral hygiene. But left unattended, it can begin in as little as eight hours after plaque has formed. All plaque does not necessarily undergo calcification, but if you are susceptible to forming calculus your plaque can become 50 percent mineralized within only two days and from 60 to 90 percent mineralized in twelve days.

Food An important distinction must be made between the type of food that causes decay and that which promotes plaque formation. Decay can only take place in the presence of sugar, while *any type of diet* will contribute to plaque formation, including a high-protein, low-fat diet or a carbohydrate-free diet. In fact, plaque formation can take place *even if no food is present*. Thus, just because you remove sugar from your diet does not mean you'll eliminate plaque, but it will help, because a soft, sticky, processed, and overcooked diet, one that is high in refined carbohydrates, is the biggest promoter of periodontal disease. In short, any food left in your mouth will contribute to plaque formation, but a diet that is high in sugar will increase the amount and rate at which plaque forms.

Saliva Saliva plays a very positive role in preventing decay and periodontal disease, but once plaque has been attached to your teeth for more than twenty-four hours, the many minerals found in saliva can contribute to the formation of calculus.

You You are the final member of the cast of characters that contribute to gum disease—or more correctly, how well or how poorly you take care of your mouth. Knowing what causes this disease will help you tremendously when it comes to preventing it. It can be very frustrating and discouraging to think you've been doing everything you should to take care of your teeth and gums, only to find that you still have the disease. Unfortunately, although you were making the effort, you didn't know how to take care of them in the right way, at the right time, and with the right tools. I include among the "tools" your relationship with the hygienist, because if you don't see her on a regular basis your disease will always be worse than if you do. Remember, if you don't know where you're going, chances are you'll never get there.

Now you that you know something about the characters in the story of periodontal disease, let's see what takes place when they appear together on the same stage, your mouth.

The Beginning: Plaque Formation

All periodontal disease begins with plaque formation. In other words, without plaque formation you wouldn't get gum disease. I should repeat that, but I won't.

Plaque is initiated when millions of disease-causing germs attach themselves to the tooth by releasing a gluelike substance. These germs can attach to what appears to the naked eye as a perfectly smooth tooth surface but, to the plaque, is actually more like a rut-filled country road. They especially love areas of the tooth that don't get cleaned properly, rough spots where decay has already started, pits and defects, and overhanging fillings. They also love the gingival crevice, the little groove where the tooth meets the gum, and the gum pocket, because these areas offer them a protected place to hang out.

But germs alone—even those that initiate plaque formation, no matter how many are attached—are not considered plaque. As more and more germs congregate, however, they're able to snag the other materials that contribute to plaque formation, such as food particles, minerals, and other germs. Once all of the ingredients have joined together—and this can occur in as little as one hour after brushing—you've officially begun to form plaque.

At this point, and up to about four hours after this sticky and nearly invisible substance has formed on your tooth's surface, the plaque is vulnerable to all forms of oral cleansing. But if you give it

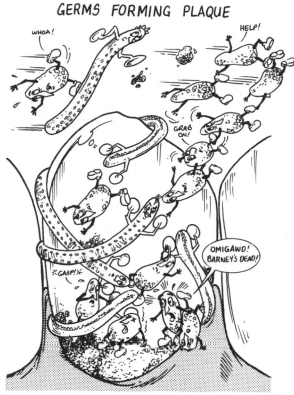

GERMS FORMING PLAQUE

more than four uninterrupted hours to establish itself, it becomes a lot tougher to remove. Left longer than that, plaque can adhere pretty solidly to the tooth, and in most cases, even brushing won't remove it all. You may scrape off the top layers, but the part that is most firmly attached to the tooth will usually remain. This makes it easier for the next layer of plaque to form, and it can begin to do so immediately after the next brushing. Remember, plaque can form in the absence of food, so even if you fast you'll still have to keep brushing.

Resisting the Plaque Invasion

As soon as the germ-laden plaque starts to form at the gum line, your body musters its defensive forces to battle the bacteria. The germs that come in contact with the gum tissue release toxins that irritate and inflame the tissue. Soon the inflammation stimulates the release of germ-fighting cells in the immediate area of the plaque formation, causing an increase of blood flow to the surface of the gum tissue, which causes the gums to swell. A battle between health and disease has now been initiated—your body's defenses versus the germs. The result is a buildup of millions of dead germs and millions of used-up, dead defense cells. As the fight continues, the battlefield debris is added to the growing plaque, and more and more plaque is formed. Once it has begun, this process goes on minute by minute, hour by hour, until you step in to have the plaque removed and to control the germ population, or until your teeth fall out. Believe me, there are better ways to overcome plaque than to lose your teeth.

Within a few days, the gums that once were firm and healthy begin to lose their tone and elasticity. As the infection proceeds, the gums lose their ability to grip the tooth firmly at the top of the gum line, and the pocket between the gum and the tooth loosens and becomes more accessible to the invasive plaque. The plaque on the teeth now spreads in all directions and begins to push into the pocket. As it does so, it comes in contact with more gum tissue, and the inflammation process expands. An ever-increasing number of your body's defensive cells are called upon to resist the germs. Without your intervention, your body's natural defenses may win a few battles, but in time they'll surely lose the war.

The Formation of Calculus

Soon, within as little as eight hours after it has begun, this massive onslaught of germ-filled plaque moves into its next phase. The portion of the plaque that lies next to the tooth begins to mineralize. You now have the beginning of calculus.

The mineralized layer of calculus bonds to the tooth even more powerfully than plaque. More plaque becomes calcified and starts to spread in all directions, pushing outward against the gum tissue, while simultaneously making its way into the extremely vul-

DR. TOM'S TIPS

It should be noted that not everyone forms calculus, and people who do form it do so at differing rates. Although calculus contributes to gum disease, you don't need to form calculus to get periodontal disease. All you need is a poor diet, poor oral hygiene, and plaque.

nerable gum pocket. New plaque is constantly being formed on top of the ever-spreading calculus.

As more gum tissue comes in contact with the spreading plaque and calculus, the infection intensifies, and the substance that holds your gum cells together is weakened. This weakening makes the gums more fragile, and soon the gums are no longer able to protect themselves even from the most mild forms of stimulation, such as brushing and eating hard foods. As a result, bleeding takes place. Once the bleeding starts, the germs get an additional source of food—the blood and other body fluids that are now being released from the gum tissue at an alarming rate. Now certain types of germs can begin to penetrate the gum tissue. This infection process is no different from what happens when you cut your finger. The germs normally found on your finger and in the air are unable to penetrate healthy, intact skin, but once the skin is cut, the invasion begins.

Bye-Bye Ligament

Once plaque begins to form in the pocket, it is protected against most forms of oral hygiene. As plaque moves into the once healthy gum pocket, the infection begins to involve the place where the ligament attaches the gum to the tooth surface. Infection here is bad enough by itself, but the whole process is made even worse by the formation of subgingival calculus. As the calculus grows and spreads, it pushes against the swollen gum tissue. The new plaque, which is continually forming on top of the expanding calculus, comes into contact with areas of gum tissue that are still healthy. When this happens the inflammation and infection spread more rapidly than ever. When the infection reaches the place where the ligament attaches the gingiva to the tooth, the ligament is forced to let go of its hold on the tooth surface, and the pocket now begins to deepen. In essence, the calculus acts as a scaffold by which the plaque gains access to the surrounding gum tissue.

How Gingivitis Becomes Periodontitis

Once the infection involves the ligament that holds the tooth to the bone, you have officially moved from gingivitis to periodontitis. As the infection destroys the ligament, both the root and the bone are exposed to the bacterial hoards and the toxins they release and to the deadly plaque and calculus. Periodontitis and root decay go hand in hand because the thin, soft layer of cementum that surrounds the root and the vulnerable dentin underneath it are directly exposed to the acid-producing germs found in the plaque.

The bone surrounding the tooth is also now at risk. The bone of the jaw is extremely susceptible to any form of irritation and infection. The bone resists this invasion on its own in the best way it knows, but without help from you, the hygienist, and the dentist, it is overwhelmed and soon has to retreat. The retreat begins when *osteoclasts*, which are cells that dissolve bone, start breaking down your jawbone to remove it from the plaque invasion and its accompanying germs and toxins. This is how *bone loss* occurs.

Prior to this stage, the battle was raging on the outer surfaces of your body; but now the battle location has moved deeper within because the first line of defense, your gums, has been breached. As the bone recedes, the pockets deepen, more plaque is formed on top of the continuously growing calculus . . . and, again, the disease process is accelerated.

Over time, as more and more bone is lost, the tooth begins to loosen. This loosening is expedited by chewing because there's not enough bone supporting the tooth to resist the tremendous forces of mastication. Eventually, the tooth becomes loose enough to be wiggled by your fingers. And the once inaccessible opening between the tooth and the gum becomes a germ superfreeway.

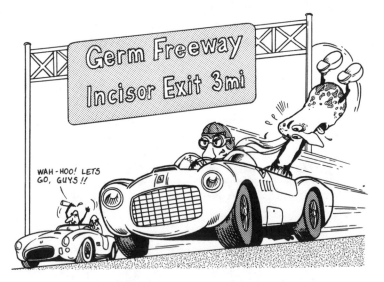

Now everything you put into your mouth has direct access to the bone, the gum tissue, and the root of the tooth. More food is packed in, more germs are born, and more plaque and calculus are formed. There is now very little you can do about it on your own. If left untreated the disease will soon pass the point of no return and it will be too late to save the tooth. Once the framework that holds the bone cells is lost to gum disease, new bone won't form to replace what has been lost, even after you get rid of the disease. At this critical stage the damage is irreversible. If the tooth is not pulled, it will eventually just fall out.

Epilogue

There you have it, the story of gum disease and how it can take a perfectly healthy tooth from your mouth on the long and painful journey to the oral surgeon's jar. If you let gum disease go too far, your story will end in the same unhappy way that it has for more than 13 million people who are now toothless.

If you're not yet concerned about this disease, you should be. Knowledge gives birth to hope and motivation, and the following chapters will give you the knowledge you need to do something about this disease. Let's begin Chapter 3 with an oral self-examination.

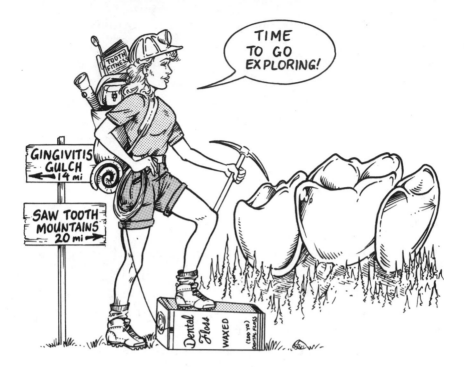

Chapter 3

Oral Self-Examination

You need to understand health before you can understand disease, so first I'll describe the look, feel, and smell of healthy gums. After that, I'll tell you how to spot the signs of gum disease, using a home method of oral self-examination. Then, in the second part of this chapter, you'll examine your teeth. And in the third part, you'll take a look at your tongue, glands, and saliva.

This self-examination is, of course, optional, but I strongly recommend that you participate. By examining your own mouth before you are professionally examined, and before you begin your new hygiene program, you'll get an invaluable baseline picture, your own visual reference point from which to monitor your progress. So write down the results of your examination; then take your results to the dental office in order to compare what you've found to what the dentist and hygienist discover.

If you repeat your home examination after spending three to four dedicated weeks on your home care program, you'll see for yourself how much can be accomplished through your own efforts. Ideally, at this point, the RDH (registered dental hygienist) will have already performed hygiene therapy, provided a lot of support and guidance, and given you your personalized instructions—but she won't have brushed, flossed, and used the water irrigator for you. Your progress will be your own, and seeing it for yourself will be motivating and empowering.

If you're one of the millions who don't regularly see a dentist this chapter will be especially important to you. Far too many people erroneously believe that if there's no pain there's no problem. This is the worst approach you can take with your teeth and is the cause of much suffering and expense. Examining your mouth will, perhaps for the first time, give you a chance to see what is actually going on in there. It's one thing to hear words like plaque, decay, gum disease, etc., and another to actually see these processes in action in your own mouth. You still may not want to do anything about them, but you can no longer use ignorance as an excuse. Use what you see to motivate you not only to get involved with your hygiene but also to get your mouth repaired.

Don't worry about missing something, because your home examination will be double-checked by the hygienist or the dentist. They'll make the official diagnosis for you. Remember, no matter how well you do on your own, you'll need the aid of the dentist and the hygienist, not only to verify what you've seen but also to pick up what you may have missed. I feel pretty confident that your self-examination will show you things you've never seen before. Are you clear about what self-examination can mean to you? Great, I like your attitude already.

WHAT YOU NEED

The tools for your self-examination are few, simple to use, easy to obtain, and inexpensive:

☐ A penlight

☐ A mouth mirror

☐ A bathroom mirror

RIGHT SIDE

LEFT SIDE

☐ Some absorbent cloth or gauze to dry the teeth and gums

☐ A good place to prop *Tooth Fitness* while you're performing your exam. You can buy a small bookstand, or you can create your own.

☐ A diagram of the teeth. The drawing above shows you the tooth numbering system the dentist and hygienist use when they communicate with each other. Whenever you find a problem area, make a note of it using this numbering system. They'll be amazed and pleased when they hear you speak of "sensitivity in number 22" versus "I have pain in the lower left side." They might even think you went to dental school.

The best way to perform your oral self-examination is with a small penlight attached to a mouth mirror. Until recently you could buy a combination mouth mirror and penlight, but it's no longer being made, so you'll have to get creative. What you need to get is a mouth mirror (Butler makes an excellent one) and a penlight (Eveready makes an inexpensive one that is perfect for this). Both can be found in most drugstores.

Mating the two is a simple procedure. Get some tape—Scotch tape works great—and place the penlight on the handle of the mouth mirror, with the bulb facing the mirror. Position it about one and one-half inches away from the mirror. Secure the penlight to the mirror handle by taping it in at least two places. Presto, you've just created a very functional hygiene tool that will serve you well, for a long time. This is the best way to do it, but if you don't want to go through this process, you can perform the examination by holding the mouth mirror in one hand and the penlight, or small flashlight, in the other hand. Place the mirror in your mouth, position it to reflect the area you want to see, and shine the light on the area. Make whatever adjustments you need to until you can see the mouth mirror reflected in the bathroom mirror. Although the mirror-light combination is easier to use, a little trial and error using them separately will provide the same results.

If the mirror fogs up, it's because the mirror is colder than your breath, but there's a way around that. Equalize the temperatures, either by running warm water over the mirror for a few seconds or by putting the mirror in your mouth and rubbing it along the inside of your cheek. The saliva will coat the mirror and keep it from fogging.

GETTING A FEEL FOR THE PROCEDURE

Before you begin the actual examination, I'd like you to get a feel for the procedure, so we'll practice viewing the gums. It's a simple technique, and after you run through it once you'll be ready to start your home examination. Don't worry about looking for anything specific at this point. You'll use the same approach to examine your teeth; so later, just replace the word *teeth* for the word *gums*. If you've got kids, this is a great way to introduce them to their mouths.

Get your equipment together, wash your hands, plant yourself firmly in front of the mirror, and as soon as you're ready, we can get down to business.

Viewing the Gums Around the Front Teeth

You don't need the mouth mirror for this part of the examination.

☐ Lean over as close to the mirror as necessary to get a good view.

☐ Place your index and middle fingers of each hand at the corner of each side of your lips and gently pry them apart. Your mouth and lips are very sensitive and delicate, so be gentle. Only separate your lips as much as necessary to clearly see.

☐ Keeping your teeth together, barely touching, move your lower jaw forward so your lower front teeth are even with the upper front teeth.

In this position you should be able to see enough of the gums around the front teeth to do the examination.

Viewing the Gums Around the Back Teeth

You have two jaws to examine, so take your pick: which one do you want to explore first? I see you chose the lower jaw. Good choice, because that's where I'm starting.

Lower jaw The gums around the outside of the lower left back teeth can be seen by taking your left index finger and pulling your lower lip out and down. In- 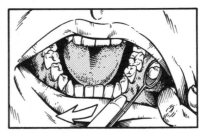 sert the mouth mirror (mirror facing toward the teeth) between the cheek and the gums. Reverse the procedure for the right side. You'll have to play with the position of the mouth mirror until you see its reflection in the bathroom mirror.

To see the gums on the inside of the lower jaw you only have to 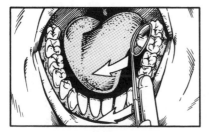 open wide enough to place the mouth mirror between the tongue and the teeth. If the tongue fights back (it can be rebellious) you can use the mouth mirror to hold it back. Tilt the mouth mirror as needed in order to see your teeth and gums reflected in the bathroom mirror. Play with it until you feel comfortable. Be sure to periodically rinse the mouth mirror with warm water if it fogs up.

Upper jaw The basics are the same. As long as you know what you're looking for, have some patience, and use your mouth mirror in the right way it'll be a breeze. Now that you're familiar with the technique, it's time to get started.

PART 1: YOUR GUMS

Healthy Gums

There are seven characteristics of healthy gums that can be observed at home. Don't flip out if your gums don't display all of the healthy signs—few do. But be honest. When your RDH examines you, she most definitely will be. Read through each description, then examine your gums and compare.

1. Healthy gums are firm. They look like someone pulled a tightly fitting spandex suit over the teeth. Think in terms of tone, as you would with muscle tone, and you'll get the idea.

2. Healthy gums are generally a pinkish color. Some may even look whitish pink. For the lower jaw, this color should extend down about one-half inch from the highest point the gum reaches on the tooth. (Reverse this for the upper jaw.) However, dark-skinned people often have healthy gums with dark pigmentation, and fair-skinned people sometimes do too, so color can't always be used as a definitive criterion. The point is: if your gums are pigmented but the remaining features check out okay, you'll know your gums are healthy.

3. Healthy gums fill in the spaces between the teeth. At the highest point between the teeth (on the lower jaw) they should be shaped like an upside down V. (Reverse this for the upper jaw.)

4. Healthy gums form a collarlike rim around the teeth. This collar, or rim, is nothing more than a roll of gum tissue that begins where the gum meets the tooth, rises up, and blends back into the gum. It's about one-sixteenth of an inch wide.

5. Healthy gums have little dotlike indentations called *stippling*. The stippling effect begins just below the collar (or above, for the upper jaw). The stippled areas should look somewhat like the skin of a naval orange.

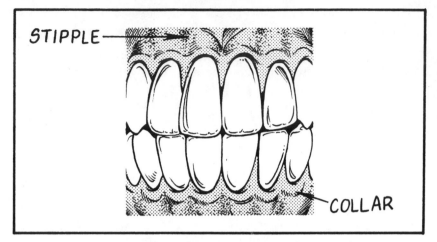

STIPPLE

COLLAR

6. Healthy gums are not tender. This also means they don't bleed when you eat or brush.

7. And finally, healthy gums are odorless. No morning, noon, or evening breath. I'm not talking about obvious breath, meaning breath that has an obvious cause (garlic, onions, cigarettes).

Unhealthy Gums

Now you know what healthy gums should look and feel like. You're also becoming more familiar with a part of your body to which you've probably never given a great deal of attention. Kind of like living next door to someone all your life and never really meeting her. It's time to see what kind of neighbors your gums are.

After you've read through the following questionnaire, which addresses the most common gum disease symptoms, I want you to examine your mouth and see how many you can find. If you think you recognize any of these symptoms, check the box and note the location. The RDH can verify it one way or another. (Please, if this book is from the library, photocopy the pages or write everything on a separate piece of paper. Thanks, from me and your librarian.) There are three boxes, one for this exam and two for additional exams, plus space for you to note the location of what you discover. Be sure to note the date of each exam.

Are your gums shiny, smooth, and without the stippled effect? To check for this, take your drying cloth and pat dry the areas that you're examining.

❏ _____

❏ _____

❏ _____

Are your gums swollen, puffy, red, and angry?

❏ _____

❏ _____

❏ _____

Do the tips of the gums (where the gums fit between the teeth) have a craterlike or hollowed-out appearance? Sort of like the recessed tip of a volcano?

❏ _____

❏ _____

❏ _____

Is there a whitish, pus-like substance at the tips of your gums? Look especially in the area of the lower front teeth.

❏ _____

❏ _____

❏ _____

Is food easily caught between any of the teeth?

❏ _____

❏ _____

❏ _____

Do your gums bleed when brushed, when eating, or at any other time, especially for no apparent reason? One good way to check for bleeding is to push on the gums with your finger in the area between the teeth.

Another way is to generate a suction effect, as if you were trying to suck the gums into your mouth between your teeth. Even if you have no bleeding at other times, but you do with this test, check the box.

❑ _____

❑ _____

❑ _____

Do you have bad breath? Dental disease (especially gum disease) and trapped food particles are the main causes of bad breath.

❑ _____

❑ _____

❑ _____

Are your gums painful? Do they feel hot or exhibit a burning sensation, as if your breath could melt snow?

❑ _____

❑ _____

❑ _____

Have the gums receded? Are there spaces between your teeth that were once filled by gums?

❑ _____

❑ _____

❑ _____

Do you have any loose teeth, or have any of your teeth shifted from their original position?

❑ _____

❑ _____

❑ _____

Is there any plaque or calculus stuck to your teeth? This is commonly seen at the gum line.

❑ _____

❑ _____

❑ _____

If you have checked a majority of the above, have you also noticed a slight fever, sore throat, loss of energy, and a general feeling of the blahs?

❑ _____

❑ _____

❑ _____

DR. TOM'S TIPS

The extent and seriousness of your gum disease will vary from area to area. You may have only the beginnings of a problem in one place and advanced disease in another. So I want you to check out your gums around every tooth, inside and out, not just the around the front teeth. When you've done this, you'll have a pretty good idea of the general condition of your gums, but you'll never know the exact condition without a full dental and oral examination.

PART 2: YOUR TEETH

While you were examining your gums you most likely saw some teeth. You'll now use the same tools and techniques to check them out. You can start the examination anywhere you want, but make sure you start and end at the same place and examine every one of your teeth. Don't brush before this examination—you're not trying to impress anyone, and I want you to see how things look before a brushing. When you examine your teeth, cover all of the following areas. If you think you have a problem check the box and note the number of the tooth or teeth involved (according to the tooth numbering system shown on page 58). Don't forget to jot down the date of your exam.

Number of Teeth

First see how many teeth you have. You should have thirty-two, counting the four wisdom teeth (if they haven't been removed).

Are you missing any teeth? Which one(s)?

❏ _____

❏ _____

❏ _____

If so, have the teeth adjacent to the missing tooth (or teeth) moved or rotated? This seems to happen most often in the lower jaw.

❏ _____

❏ _____

❏ _____

If you have a missing tooth, has the tooth above, or below, the empty space moved into the void? You can check this by closing your mouth as you would normally, and then, with your fingers, separating your lips; see if the tooth above (or below) the missing one has moved into the empty space. You might have to use your mouth mirror to see this.

❏ _____

❏ _____

❏ _____

If the tooth has moved, your situation is serious; some of the tooth may have to be removed or crowned to make room for the false tooth. But whether it's moved or not, you'll have to replace the missing tooth or you'll probably end up losing the opposing tooth. Whenever you lose a tooth, the opposing tooth no longer functions while you are chewing, and, in effect, you lose both of them. For example, if you keep your lower teeth but lose all your uppers, you lose the function of all thirty-two because the bottoms can't function without the tops.

Shape and Size

Judging by the wide variety of sizes and shapes found in nature, I'd say that God or Nature isn't too concerned with creating everyone alike. Statistics show that the so-called perfect mouth, dentally speaking, is found in only 2 percent of the population. A tooth that is misshapen, too small, or too large will usually not be a problem for your dental health. As far as aesthetics are concerned, however, it could be. Cosmetic dentistry (see Chapter 13) can do wonders to correct a problem tooth, so make a note of its location and point it out to your dentist.

Are any of your teeth candidates for cosmetic dentistry?

❑ _____

❑ _____

❑ _____

Spaces between Your Teeth

There are natural and unnatural spaces found between the teeth. Most natural ones won't cause a problem—they're usually wide enough so that most food won't get stuck in between them—and other than your own feelings about them aesthetically, they're nothing to be concerned about. In chil- TEETH 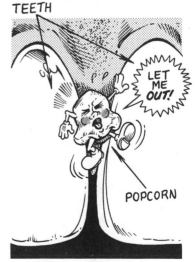 dren it's actually normal and desirable to have these spaces in order for there to be enough room for the proper emergence of the permanent teeth.

Unnatural spaces are another story entirely. These spaces—and I'm not speaking about the spaces caused by lost teeth—are more easily felt or experienced than seen. For example, if after eating certain types of fibrous, tough, or stringy foods—like meat, oranges, popcorn—you feel some-

LET ME OUT!

POPCORN

thing stuck between your teeth that even a good brushing won't remove, you can be pretty sure that you've located an unnatural space. It may feel like the food is stuck in the gums or wedged between the two teeth. In the dental profession the place where two teeth touch is called a *contact point.* "Bad contacts" or "poor contacts"—where the contacts aren't as tight as they should be—can be caused by decay, a broken filling, or a poorly designed or placed filling. No matter how it's caused, an unnatural space is going to end up causing you some serious gum problems. Because food that gets stuck can't be removed by brushing, these areas are very susceptible to decay and gum disease. They must be fixed. Until you do, make sure you floss immediately after you eat.

Do you have any unnatural spaces between your teeth? Note location.

❏ _____

❏ _____

❏ _____

Overlapped (Crowded) and Rotated Teeth

If only 2 percent of us have perfectly straight teeth that means you have a 98 percent chance of having at least one tooth that isn't. Aside from genetics, lost teeth are the most common cause of this problem. Teeth that are too far out of normal alignment can cause one or more of the following problems:

☐ They're more difficult to keep clean.

☐ They can interfere with your bite and with normal chewing.

☐ They can cause *temporomandibular joint* (TMJ) problems.

☐ They can be unsightly.

☐ Children's permanent teeth may come in improperly.

If you can afford it, there's much that can be done through orthodontic treatment and cosmetic dentistry. If you choose not to go that route, or you can't afford orthodontic treatment, you can still keep them healthy by knowing how to take care of overlapped or rotated teeth.

Do you have any teeth that aren't properly aligned? Note the location because you'll need to spend extra time keeping them healthy.

❏ _____

❏ _____

❏ _____

Malocclusion and TMJ Problems

There are a surprising number of people, whether they're aware of it or not, who have at least some problems resulting from *malocclusion*, or a bad bite. Bite problems can range from minor ones involving only an improperly placed filling (easily corrected), to those caused by lost teeth, to genetic ones (overcrowding and jaw misalignment) involving most or all your teeth.

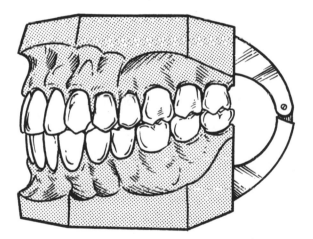

Is your bite even? A simple way to test this is to swallow and then immediately lightly tap your teeth together. If the sound is an evenly distributed "tap, tap" or "clunk, clunk," you should be fine. You can also use your mouth mirror to check this. Bite down, insert the mouth mirror, pull your lips apart, and see if the teeth come together as shown in the drawing. Note any differerences.

❏ _____

❏ _____

❏ _____

Bite down slowly (without food in your mouth). Are you hitting on one side of your jaws before the other? To test this, relax your jaw muscles as much as possible, swallow, and your teeth will come together naturally. Don't try to guide your lower jaw closed. Think about something else, so your mind doesn't get too involved, and let your mouth close naturally.

❏ _____

❏ _____

❏ _____

Again, closing slowly, does it feel as if you're hitting on just one tooth, or a filling, first? This is subtle, so pay attention. You may notice that instead of hitting evenly on all the teeth's surfaces at once you first hit on one tooth and then the rest of the teeth slide into place.

❏ _____

❏ _____

❏ _____

Do your teeth, or some of them, feel sore for no apparent reason, and are they especially tender during or after chewing?

❏ _____

❏ _____

❏ _____

If you have difficulty opening your jaw fully this could be an indication of a *temporomandibular joint* (TMJ) disorder. This disorder, marked by pain and discomfort in the jaw joint, affects millions of people. It's most often caused by prolonged tooth clenching or grinding; a bad bite; injury to the joint, ligaments, or muscles; genetics; or a degeneration of the bone or the ligaments of the jaw joint. It could also be caused by a wisdom tooth impaction or extraction. If you have any of the following symptoms you may have a TMJ problem.

Are the muscles in the general area where the lower jaw hinges with the upper jaw sore, tired, or tense?

❑ _____

❑ _____

❑ _____

Can you hear a cracking, clicking, or popping sound when you open your mouth to talk, yawn, or chew?

❑ _____

❑ _____

❑ _____

Does your lower jaw slide out of its socket (or almost do so) when you open wide?

❑ _____

❑ _____

❑ _____

Check the tops of your teeth. Are there any wear spots, either on your fillings or on your natural tooth surfaces? Check especially the place where you seem to hit first when you bite down. These high spots will appear shiny if there's a filling, or worn if it's the natural tooth. If you have a very serious problem you'll see that your cusp tips are worn down.

❑ _____

❑ _____

❑ _____

It is very important to verify any suspicions you have about a bite or TMJ problem with your dentist. Most of these bite problems begin as simple ones and become complex through neglect. They not only can cause nutritional problems (by forcing you to change to a softer, less natural diet) but may also lead to severe bone loss. If the problem is caught early enough it can easily be corrected, but if you let it go the problem could become very serious, and at that point the average dentist may not be able to offer you a simple and inexpensive solution. You could thus end up paying an unnecessary, heavy price for delaying its treatment.

Serious bite and TMJ problems are among the least understood aspects of dentistry. If it has been determined that you have an advanced condition ask your dentist to refer you to a dentist who specializes in TMJ problems. I suggest you don't let anyone experiment with you unless he specializes in these areas and promises to get results. Asking him to commit to the outcome is one way of making him think twice before he uses you as a guinea pig.

Stains and Discolorations

It's easy for the layperson to confuse a stain with decay, but most stains have an external cause and are generally harmless, though they can be an eyesore. You can also mistake a stain for the discoloration caused by an amalgam filling, which can darken the surrounding tooth structure. Normally, routine hygiene therapy will remove self-imposed stains, but if any stain remains after the cleaning have the dentist check it out.

Stains come in all colors and can be caused by many things, most of which aren't good for you.

Natural discoloration Most teeth start out bluish white when you're young and get yellow to grayish yellow as you get older. So if you used to have white teeth and they're now yellow, don't panic. You may just be facing the thing most of us try to avoid—the normal aging process. The white part of your teeth, the enamel, gets worn away with age, and because it's somewhat transparent, the more the enamel is worn off, the more the yellow-colored dentin found directly under the enamel shows through.

This is a normal process, unless the enamel wears off too rapidly. For example, if you're thirty years old and your teeth were white one month and yellow the next month, you may have a problem. Rapid wearing of the enamel can be caused by any number of factors: genetically soft enamel, an abrasive diet, a highly acidic mouth, an acidic diet (are you sucking on lemons, drinking acidic soft

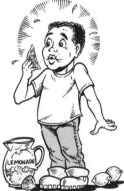

drinks?), rare diseases, overuse of an abrasive or acidic toothpaste, or a potentially harmful work environment (like a sandblasting company). Whew!

Have you observed that your teeth are yellowing too fast? If so, you and your dentist should do a Sherlock Holmes and ascertain the cause. Once the cause is known you have a chance to correct it.

❏ _____

❏ _____

❏ _____

Green stains　Green stains are most often found on children's teeth, usually at or around the point where the teeth and gums meet, most obviously on the front teeth. The stain is actually on the membrane that covers the erupting tooth. Normally the membrane is sloughed off during the eruption process. If it isn't, a simple cleaning should remove it.

Did you find any green stains?

❏ _____

❏ _____

❏ _____

Brown stains　Brown stains are usually caused by smoking or by chewing tobacco. They can also be caused by drinking a lot of coffee or tea. But the major contributor is poor oral hygiene. What? Well, these substances will more readily stain plaque and calculus than your teeth. Many people think their teeth are stained when it is actually the plaque and/or calculus that is stained.

So look closely. Do you have this type of stain on the portion of the teeth closest to the gum line?

❏ _____

❏ _____

❏ _____

Dark gray, yellow, brown, or black stains   These are discolorations that you should look for not only in your own teeth but also in your child's. They usually indicate that the pulp (the portion of the tooth containing the nerves and blood vessels) is dying or has died. It can be the result of decay. Or it can be from a blow to the tooth (usually it's the front teeth that are involved). It doesn't have to be a powerful shot to the tooth to kill it. A well-placed blow will cause the blood vessels in the pulp to hemorrhage; the blood then leaks into the pulp cavity and into the tubules in the dentin. The resulting dark dentin shows through the transparent enamel and—walla!—you have a discolored tooth. The discoloration won't show up immediately; so if you fell off a horse last week, ran into a wall, or were hit by a baseball, forgot about it after the pain subsided, and now have a discolored tooth, you can put two and two together. If you're a parent you know that kids are always taking weird falls, so be sure to watch for this.

Have any of your teeth become discolored over a short period of time?

❏ _____

❏ _____

❏ _____

White or brown chalky spots   An excessive intake of fluoride during the formation of the crowns of the teeth can cause discolorations. Although this is somewhat unsightly, you won't find decay in those areas. You can read more about the fluoride issue in Chapter 18.

Do you have any chalky stains?

❏ _____

❏ _____

❏ _____

Decay

We've already discussed tooth decay and the areas where it is most often found. (If you want to refresh your memory, turn back to pages 34–36 in Chapter 1.) When you examine your teeth always look closely in these areas. Usually there will be discoloration and a flaw, or hole, in the enamel or root.

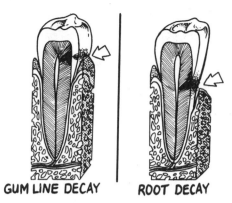

GUM LINE DECAY   ROOT DECAY

Do you see anything that looks like decay?

❑ _____

❑ _____

❑ _____

Broken or Lost Fillings

All restorations can wear down, fracture (except gold), or fall out. Check the margins around every filling to see if they're intact, especially those on the tooth's chewing surfaces.

Are any of your fillings worn down, broken, or missing?

❑ _____

❑ _____

❑ _____

Broken, Chipped, or Cracked Teeth

Broken and chipped teeth are easy to find. If you see a tooth that doesn't look normal check its twin on the opposite side. If it doesn't match up you should make note of that tooth. Keep in mind that a tooth can break or chip without giving pain, so unless you examine your teeth, it may go unnoticed. Look especially hard at the front teeth and at teeth where you have experienced any sensitivity to heat, cold, acidic substances, and, especially, sugar-containing foods or snacks.

Do you have any broken, chipped, or cracked teeth?

❏ _____

❏ _____

❏ _____

Cracks and fractures are often too small to see with the naked eye. It will be much easier to spot them if you dry the teeth before you start looking. Most often a crack in a tooth will be noticed more by feeling than by sight. You wake up early one day, walk outside, take a mouth full of refreshingly cool morning air, and feel a pain in number 9. Or, lord forbid, you eat a candy bar and soon feel a sharp twinge of pain, or even a little twinge, in number 29. If this happens be sure you make note of it, because the dentist may not see the fracture unless you tell him, and it could, so to speak, slip through the cracks.

Have you noticed any area of pain, or sensitivity, in a tooth that shows no other signs of disease?

❏ _____

❏ _____

❏ _____

Erosion and Abrasion

These terms simply mean that your teeth are being abnormally worn away by various substances that probably have no business being in your mouth in the first place. Erosion and abrasion are much easier to feel than to see. A dramatic way of detecting them is to visit the RDH. When she starts poking around with her little metal explorer and she touches one or more of those eroded or abraded areas, you may immediately feel a sensation that can only be described as shocking. Don't tough it out. Tell her immediately. Unless your scream provided her with the information she needed.

Erosion   Erosion is abnormal wear due a chemical reaction. A good example of an erosion-causing agent is the lemon. Lemons, as well as other citrus fruit, contain natural acids that are strong enough to completely dissolve the tooth's enamel and dentin, given a long enough period of time. This process is akin to a river's effect on rocks. Of course it happens much faster in your mouth, especially if you're a heavy lemon sucker and also have soft teeth.

Have your gums receded, showing more of the tooth than before, although you don't have gum disease? What's happening is that acid is etching away the tooth and chemically detaching the ligaments that connect the gum to the tooth. If you have exposed roots you will be more vulnerable to both erosion and abrasion, so be sure and check out these areas.

❏ _____

❏ _____

❏ _____

Are your teeth sensitive to heat or cold, sweets, or brushing at the gum line?

❏ _____

❏ _____

❏ _____

If you can't break the lemon habit you can at least rinse well immediately after sucking on one, or juice the lemon and drink it through a straw and then rinse. Other acidic substances may also cause erosion, with the basic symptoms being the same. For example, take the phosphoric acid that is normally found in many types of soft drinks. This acid is strong enough to dissolve an iron nail—so what chance have your teeth got? Combine this acid with the approximately four and one-half teaspoons of sugar found in a twelve-ounce bottle of some soft drinks and you have more than enough to cause not only erosion but also decay. Soft drinks and candy have probably decayed more teeth than all other foods and drinks combined. Just imagine if you drank a lot of soft drinks, ate a lot of candy, and also sucked on lemons. Whew! Do you have dental insurance?

Many times the sensitivity stemming from erosion can be corrected by simply finding and eliminating the cause. There are also a few special kinds of toothpastes that can help treat it. If the problem has gone too far your dentist can desensitize the area with any one of the many desensitizing methods available to him; or you can have fillings placed in the sensitive areas, as a last resort.

Abrasion Abrasion is like erosion—the tooth is being worn away—but the cause is mechanical rather than chemical. Abrasive sandpaper rubbing on soft wood will abrade the wood very rapidly. Same goes for the teeth, except the cause, I hope, won't be sandpaper. The rate of wear will depend on the strength of your enamel, the abrasiveness of the material, and how often you use it.

The end result is very similar to that of erosion, so look for the same symptoms and signs, but look for a different cause. Abrasion can be caused by a surprising variety of activities.

BRUSHING THE WRONG WAY I've seen cases where incorrect brushing, a side-to-side motion instead of an up-and-down rotary motion, has worn teeth in half. The teeth looked as if they were sandblasted. The effects of wrong-way brushing will be compounded if the toothpaste is an abrasive one, you use a hard-bristled toothbrush, you brush often and with a lot of force, and if all of this is done over a long period of time.

TOOTHPICKS When the toothpick is pushed in and out of the spaces between the teeth, it not only pushes the gum downward (or upward, depending on whether you're working on the lower or upper teeth), but also acts like a piece of sandpaper on the thin part of the enamel near the gum line. Eventually, this procedure will push the gum past where it normally attaches. When this happens, the toothpick will begin to abrade the root, creating toothpick

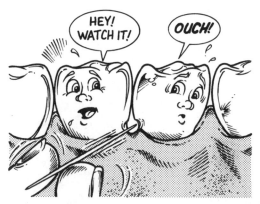

"craters." If you have any bone loss this process will be accelerated. As well as being unsightly and increasing tooth sensitivity, these craters are food traps. Used correctly, toothpicks can be an effective tool, but if you see any signs of toothpick abrasion you'll have to lighten up. (Its proper use is discussed in Chapter 5, on home care.)

Examine the areas where you use a toothpick the most. Do you detect any abrasion or gum recession?

❏ _____

❏ _____

❏ _____

THREAD AND HAIRPIN BITING If you use your teeth to break thread or open hairpins, the effects are very easy to spot, especially on the edges of the upper front teeth. That seemingly small notch you have created can set up a fracture line in the tooth, and if the notch is hit in the right way it can fracture or crack the tooth. The best treatment is to stop using your teeth for these purposes and to have the dentist smooth and polish the notched areas.

Do you have any notches on your teeth?

❏ _____

❏ _____

❏ _____

SEED SHUCKING If you love sunflower seeds, pumpkin seeds, or any others (the way I do), eat a lot of them (the way I do), and shuck them with your front teeth (the way I used to), you can wear away the enamel of the front teeth and set up fracture lines on their chewing edges. Use your back teeth instead; they're better suited for the task.

Do you have any irregularities on the edges of your front teeth? Ask the dentist to smooth them off.

❏ _____

❏ _____

❏ _____

CLENCHING AND BRUXISM Severe clenching and bruxism (grinding) can actually flex the tooth at the junction where the enamel meets the root. This may cause sensitivity.

Are the tops of your teeth are excessively worn? Are your chewing muscles always sore. Do you have pain in the TMJ joints? If you do and have tooth sensitivity be sure to tell your dentist.

❏ _____

❏ _____

❏ _____

PART 3: YOUR TONGUE, GLANDS, AND SALIVA

No self-examination would be complete without taking a peek at some of the other parts of your mouth besides teeth and gums. As with your teeth and gums, this exploration is only meant to help you become better acquainted with your mouth—to check things out and become aware of where they're found and what is normal—but by no means should you attempt to make a final diagnosis. If you find something that seems suspicious, bring it to the attention of your hygienist and dentist.

The Tongue

You might think that the tongue is best used for sticking out at someone or for kissing. If that's what you think, you're only partly right. The tongue also serves you in many more practical ways. In fact, it's one of the most interesting and observable organs of your body. Let's take a look at it before I tell you what it can do for you.

Examine your tongue Get a small piece of clean cloth or a four-by-four-inch piece of gauze. Stick out your tongue and fold the cloth over the protruding tip, then hold it out. Be firm but gentle; the tongue is a slippery little bugger and doesn't seem to like leaving its den. The cloth or gauze will help keep it in line. If you're a person with a strong will, you might try to skip the gauze and order it to do as it's told. Give it a try. But remember, it's an organ that normally acts on its own. While you have your tongue out, examine the following characteristics:

SIZE AND SHAPE   The size and shape of the tongue varies from individual to individual. I've always thought tongues were as unique as fingerprints because I've never seen two alike.

The tongue has the unique ability to change its size and shape. It can grow or shrink, depending on the conditions. For example, if you lost your teeth and didn't have them replaced, the tongue would grow larger and try to fill all of the new available space. (I guess you could say that one of the unsung achievements of your teeth is keeping your tongue in place.) And it's so adaptable that when you have your teeth replaced, your tongue will eventually shrink back to the space God gave it in the first place. This shrinking process normally takes a few months.

The shape of your tongue is a reflection of your jaws and genetic heritage. Though I've seen many shapes, I've yet to see a forked one . . .

COLOR AND COATING   Another aspect of this snakelike organ is its color and its coating. Some theorists believe the tongue's appearance means absolutely nothing, while others believe it can be a mirror of your entire digestive system and a good indicator of your general state of health. Personally, I subscribe to the latter theory. It has been aptly said that the eyes are the window of the soul, and I wholeheartedly agree, but I would add that the tongue is the window of the body.

The color and the thickness of the coating vary from day to day and can range from a fiery reddish purple, to a calm and healthy-looking pink or light red, to a pasty white and gray. You can also have a mixture of the reddish color and the pasty coating. The most important thing to know is that a healthy tongue has no bumps, lumps, open sores, ulcers, abnormal swellings, major discolorations, or pain.

Does your tongue have any lumps, sores, ulcers, swellings, discolorations? Does it give you pain? If so, have your dentist check it out.

❏ _____

❏ _____

❏ _____

What the tongue does for you This fascinating muscle organ is absolutely necessary for many of the functions we take for granted. It is especially important for maintaining our oral health. See if you were aware of the following:

- ☐ It's the principle organ of taste, and this is an excellent reason to keep it clean. If it's heavily coated your sense of taste will be reduced. This generally leads people to an unnecessary, and possibly unhealthy, increase in the use of salt, spices, and seasonings.

- ☐ It's invaluable when it comes to talking. Hold it still and try talking. See what I mean?

- ☐ It moves food around the mouth as you are chewing, mixing and shifting it from one side of the jaw to the other so that you don't overwork the teeth on just one side. You can consciously experience this movement by focusing on your chewing. Don't try to control anything, just feel what happens as your tongue moves from side to side.

- ☐ It's the main mover of food to the back of the throat so that it can be swallowed.

- ☐ It's one of the most sensual parts of our bodies. I'll say no more about this—it's better left to your own imagination—except to add that it deserves to be treated better, if only for that reason.

- ☐ It's a decay fighter. While chewing, talking, or just having fun, the tongue helps to clean the teeth and massage the gums. You can consciously take advantage of this ability by moving it around the teeth and gums, especially when you find it impossible to brush, floss, or rinse after eating.

Now that you're more aware of its value, you can treat it a little better. In Chapter 5, I'll discuss how to do just that.

The Salivary Glands

Have you ever thought about the role your salivary glands play? Do you know where they're located? No? Well, you're not alone, because most people don't. Though you don't have to be a student of them, you ought to know a few things about them.

There are four of these glands in your mouth. Two *mandibular salivary glands* are found under your tongue, directly behind and below your lower front teeth. You would be right on target if you stuck your (clean) index finger over your lower front four teeth and gently pushed it down and back until you touched what feels like soft skin. This is also the area where the tongue is attached, and once your finger is there you can wiggle your tongue slightly. This will confirm that you are right on top of the mandibular salivary glands.

The other two glands are located in the cheeks, one on each side, almost directly opposite the upper last two molars. These are called *maxillary salivary glands*, and they're are a little harder to see. Take a good look, and if you notice two little sacklike projections in that area you've found them. However, it is nice to know that even if you can't find them, they're still there and working for you.

These little spit glands are very sensitive, and if bruised or damaged in any way they can become very tender and even painful. The area around the irritated gland will feel as if you have a small piece of leather hanging there. The lower gland is particularly susceptible, so be careful when you brush in this area, bite on hard substances with your front teeth, or use a water irrigation device.

Are you having any tenderness around your salivary glands? Which one?

☐ _____

☐ _____

☐ _____

Though relatively rare, you may encounter another problem—plugged salivary glands. This is caused by stonelike objects created either by the mineralization of saliva or by disease. They are somewhat like gallstones or kidney stones. As they grow in size they block the opening into the mouth; the saliva is trapped and the gland swells up. If this happens you will both see and feel it, as it can become quite painful. This condition can happen to any of the three glands and you'll recognize the problem by the location and the pain. If you think this is happening to you make an emergency appointment with your dentist or an oral surgeon.

Saliva

The consistency of the saliva can vary from person to person and from one time of the day to another. It can range from a light, watery consistency to a heavy, ropy, mucous consistency, changing with the conditions in which you find yourself. If you are dehydrated your saliva is reduced and is thicker, reflecting your increased need for liquids. The flow of saliva is also reduced if you're nervous, angry, or afraid. The best indicator of general health and the most effective decay-fighting saliva is the watery kind.

Check the consistency of your saliva. Is it thick and syrupy? So much so that you have a hard time spitting? Or is it dry or foamy, and does it seem as if you don't have enough?

❏ _____

❏ _____

❏ _____

The benefits of saliva Saliva lubricates and allows us to swallow our food. The tongue may be the forklift that delivers food to the throat, but without the saliva it would never get to its ultimate destination. Ever try swallowing food when you don't have any saliva?

☐ Saliva acts as a chemical buffer: it has the unique ability to neutralize things that end up in your mouth that may be too acidic or too basic. This is critical when it comes to neutralizing the acid produced by decay-causing germs. If the saliva is too thick, however, it cannot effectively penetrate the germ-filled plaque.

☐ Saliva helps disinfect your mouth, on a small scale, and helps heal wounds and cuts that occur in the mouth. Along with the acid buffers, the saliva contains minerals, enzymes, germ-fighting cells, and a few other guardians that help keep the peace.

The bad news Except for a few blessed souls, nothing on this planet is perfect. Such, too, is the case with saliva, because there are two ways it can do harm.

1. Saliva is high in minerals. That alone isn't a bad thing, but if you leave plaque around too long the minerals in the saliva will turn the plaque into calculus.

2. The second major problem associated with saliva is a disease called *xerostomia*. (This is a great Scrabble word.) This condition, the inability to produce saliva, is relatively rare in its pure form, but it can occur to lesser degrees in many people. Most of us have temporarily experienced it as "dry mouth" or "cotton mouth." If you've ever had it, you have a general idea of what this disease is about—only the victim of this disease has it all the time. This condition, even in its milder forms, should be treated, because it not only creates problems with speech, digestion, and swallowing but also drastically increases the incidence of decay and other oral infections.

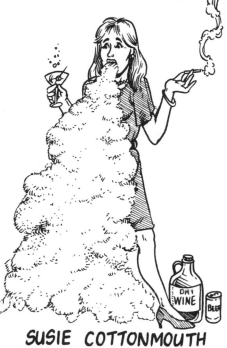

SUSIE COTTONMOUTH

Are you experiencing "dry mouth"? If it persists for one to two weeks, or more, and there doesn't seem to be any obvious reason for it (like being scared out of your boots), make an appointment to see your dentist.

❏ _____

❏ _____

❏ _____

In general, the healthier you are, the healthier your saliva will be. Make sure you drink a lot of water and cut down on your consumption of alcoholic beverages, because alcohol is a diuretic and causes dehydration.

OTHER DISEASES OF THE MOUTH

Although it's true that dental disease is the most prevalent oral disease with which you must contend, it isn't the only one, nor is it the most serious one. There are many types of cancers, growths, and abnormal skin conditions that involve the mouth. Every year nearly thirty thousand people are diagnosed with oral cancer. If the cancer is caught early, the five-year survival rate is 90 percent. If not, it drops to 50 percent. Prevention . . . prevention . . . prevention!

You may have eliminated tooth and gum disease, and your hygiene therapy visits may have been reduced to one per year, but cancer and other diseases that show up in the mouth won't follow your recall schedule. This makes performing your periodic oral exam doubly important—your own exam could reveal a potential problem much earlier than your recall exam.

The two main reasons that oral cancers are so difficult to detect early are (1) many people don't have regular dental exams, and (2) most people never examine themselves. Have you ever—before now—examined yourself for oral cancer? That's what I thought. I'll admit that it's much easier to see something on your hand than on your gums, your tongue, or on the inside of your cheek, but if you ever get an oral cancer you'll wish that you'd taken a few moments to do an exam. Don't—*ever*—hold back from pointing out something that you think might be abnormal because you don't want your dentist or RDH to think you're silly or a hypochondriac.

After you've had your dental exam and it's been determined that you're free from any oral disease, you'll know what a normal, healthy mouth looks like. Make sure you imprint that picture in your mind's eye. It'll be your reference point. I recommend that you give your oral cavity a quick check for diseases at least once a month. You don't have to know the name of what you find—just that it isn't normal, where it is, and when you first noticed it.

Pull your lips back, use the mouth mirror and light, and give your mouth a once-over. If something strange has appeared with no obvious cause, and it doesn't disappear within two weeks, call for an appointment. This applies even if it's something you think you recognize, like herpes or cold sores.

Although you may not be able to prevent these diseases from occurring in your mouth, you can definitely catch them early. To do this, you should know the six warning signs of oral cancer:

1. An ulceration, redness, or sore spot on the lips, tongue, or inside of the mouth that does not heal itself within two weeks

2. Swelling of the lips, gums, or other areas of the mouth, face, and neck

3. White scaly areas inside the mouth

4. Recurrent bleeding, with no apparent cause

5. Loss of feeling (numbness) in any part of your tongue, lips, or oral cavity

6. Persistent coughing or difficulty in swallowing or speaking

Because most people aren't aware of just how many kinds of cancers and other diseases are found in the mouth (or show signs and symptoms there), I've listed twenty-five of them. There are more, but this list should make it dramatically apparent that dental disease isn't the only oral disease you must be on the lookout for.

Abnormal bone growth	Leukemia
Abnormal soft tissue growth	Leukoplakia
AIDS	Malignant melanoma
Canker sore	Myoblastoma
Drug reaction	Nevus
Epilepsy	Nutritional deficiency
Fibroma	Papilloma
Hairy tongue	Skin disorder
Hemangioma	Squamous cell carcinoma
Hemophilia	Syphilis
Herpes	Thrush
Idiopathic disease (unknown cause)	Tuberculosis
Kaposi's sarcoma	

SOMETHING TO THINK ABOUT

It's not within the scope of this book to teach you how to diagnose or treat any of the many oral diseases that can show up in your mouth. It takes years of training to be able to do that, and treatment is updated regularly. This isn't the time to play Dr. Kildare—leave the diagnosis and treatment up to your dentist or doctor. We're not just talking about saving a tooth here, we're talking about your life.

All right. You've just learned a ton of stuff. You definitely know more about your mouth than you did thirty-three pages ago. I know this was a long chapter, but this information will serve you well.

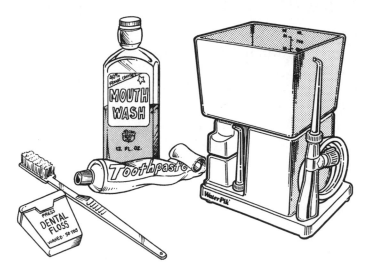

Chapter 4

The Tools of Your Trade

You are about to become a specialist in preventive dental hygiene. Like any specialist, you need to be thoroughly knowledgeable about your tools. You need to know which tools are available and how to pick the best tools for your unique oral condition. How and when you use these tools will be an important part of a successful preventive program.

WHY USE TOOLS?

Sadly, the changes that have occurred so rapidly in our modern diet have not been as kind to our mouths and bodies as the more natural diet of the past. It has taken us a long time to understand the dental health problems these changes have created. We are finally realizing that if we can no longer prevent tooth and gum disease by consuming a natural diet we must somehow make up for what nature once freely provided. Therefore you need to know everything you can about the tools that replace the cleansing action of a natural diet. Your present diet and the extent of your dental disease will together determine which tools you need to cure your dental disease and prevent future disease.

THE FREE TOOLS

The following will certainly not be considered tools in the classic sense, but without them, the store-bought ones will be like pictures on the wall—only nice to look at.

Time

This could be easily the single most important tool at your disposal. Also, it's free and needs no maintenance. Without the willingness to commit your time, the quality and number of your preventive tools won't matter at all.

Hands

These are also free. If you want to get rid of nasty gum and tooth disease you'll have to convince your hands to go to work. At first you may have to be patient with them. Making the necessary eye-to-brain and brain-to-hand connections can be awkward in the beginning—but don't worry, in a few weeks your hands will act as if they've always been performing preventive hygiene. Once you get them programmed, it will be a breeze. Your commitment to change your old patterns must be firm if you don't want to continue down the same old dental disease path.

Diet

The only completely natural way to clean your teeth is with your diet. Every other tool you use was invented because most of us haven't taken advantage of this natural tool as much as we should. By diet, I mean disease-preventing foods, not disease-causing ones. If you're willing to use more of these natural tools you'll need fewer of the mechanical ones. A natural diet is described in Chapter 16.

TRADITIONAL DENTAL TOOLS

The Toothbrush

There are over seventy different kinds of toothbrushes, with new ones appearing constantly. Toothbrushes come in all sizes, shapes, stiffness, and colors. The condition of your mouth will dictate which kind of brush will be best. For example, the type of brush you use during the initial treatment stage of your preventive program may not be the same type you'll use for the maintenance stage. Also, you may find that you need more than one kind of brush to care for different areas of your mouth. The information you obtain from this book and your hygienist will help you decide which brushes you need. Here are the main points to consider when purchasing your toothbrush.

Stiffness of the bristles Most brushes come with hard, medium, or soft bristles. For people with periodontal disease, the general rule is to use a soft-bristle brush until the disease is eliminated and a soft or medium one for maintenance. Personally, I do not recommend hard-bristle brushes while you're treating periodontal disease. The bristles of most hard brushes are not flexible enough to bend into the gingival crevice, and if used incorrectly, or with too much force, they can cause more harm than good to the tender and diseased gum tissue. When your gums have healed and can withstand the contact with hard bristles you may then want to change to a hard-bristle brush.

Hard-bristle brushes are valuable when you've missed a few brushings and want to give your teeth some extra scouring action; however, you could also use a medium brush with baking soda to get the same results, but with less trauma to the gums.

I know of no industry rules standardizing the stiffness of toothbrush bristles. One brand of hard-bristle brushes may be harder than another brand. Therefore, be tuned in when you choose a brush, and switch to a softer or harder brush if you or your hygienist feel you should.

Composition of bristles There are two kinds of bristles available—natural and synthetic. I suggest that you try both and decide for yourself which you like better.

Natural-bristle toothbrushes are made in fewer sizes, shapes, and stiffnesses. They are also more difficult to find; your local health food store is the best place to look for them. Because they are porous, natural bristles need more time to dry out in order to retain their normal stiffness. So if you decide on a natural-bristle toothbrush, keep two of them around: one for the morning and one for the evening. This gives each toothbrush twenty-four hours to dry. Over time these bristles will fray at the ends, and some dentists feel this is an advantage because there will be more bristles working for you. Most natural bristles are made from boar hair.

Synthetic-bristle toothbrushes generally have bristles made of nylon. These brushes are much easier to find and come in greater variety. Now, more and more toothbrush manufacturers are rounding the ends of the bristles during the manufacturing process, the theory being that rounded tips won't irritate gums while you are brushing. Some professionals feel that this is an advantage, albeit on a microscopic level. I think that rounded bristles are a nice touch, but not necessary for maintaining dental health.

Regardless of the type of bristle you select, a toothbrush will only do for you what you do with it.

Size To choose the best size, consider the size of your mouth. The smaller and narrower your mouth and dental arch, the smaller the brush's head and handle should be. Don't judge your mouth's size by your body size: you can have a large body and a small mouth!

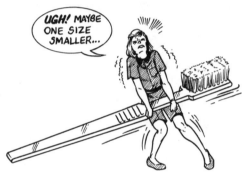

The right-size toothbrush gives you better control and better access and therefore does a much better job. For adults, the length of the bristle portion should be somewhere in the three-quarter-to-one-inch range. You don't have to bring a tape measure to the store with you, however, to check the length—just use your thumb as a guide (it's about one inch at its widest point). You may be tempted to buy a brush with a longer row of bristles, thinking you'll cover more ground with each stroke. A longer brush may work fine for the outsides of the teeth, but it makes it almost impossible to effectively brush the insides of the front teeth and the backsides of the last molars. Always keep in mind that it's not the speed or size of the boat that counts but how well you can sail it. Be brave. Experiment. But be sure to let the results of your brushing be your final guide. If your RDH keeps telling you that there are areas you're not reaching, you may have to change brush sizes or get an additional, different-size brush for problem areas. If she recommends that you change to another type of toothbrush, or that you add any other dental tool, be sure to take her advice.

A few more details. The overall length of the toothbrush should be about seven inches. You have many handle shapes and sizes from which to choose: angled ones, thick and thin ones. Select one that feels comfortable. Ideally, your brush should have between seven and thirteen rows of bristles the long way and three to four rows across. Finding a brush with the number of rows in this range is important because it allows enough flexibility to give you access to the gingival crevice without having to force too many bristles into the crevice. I use the Butler G·U·M line of toothbrushes. Butler makes the largest selection, both for adults and children, and their brushes can be found in most drugstores and supermarkets.

If you are a parent or guardian you should know a lot more about taking care of your child's teeth than how to choose the appropriate toothbrush, and Chapter 17 gives specific information about child care. As for choosing a toothbrush, the rule for adults applies as well to children: the size of the mouth determines the size of the brush. Just make sure it isn't too big. Unless your dentist or hygienist tells you differently, use a soft children's brush when you brush a child's teeth, and change to a larger one when all the baby teeth have been replaced by permanent ones.

Shape The straight, standard, average, old-fashioned brush is just fine—but only if you use it in the right way. If you use a brush specifically designed to work in a particular area it may not be as effective in other areas. For example, a curved brush will work well in curved areas, but it isn't very effective in flat areas or where the curve is reversed. The standard-shape brush is the most universal, but without you to guide it, no brush will work.

Specially shaped brushes You only need to use specially shaped brushes if you have one or more of the following conditions:

- ☐ Missing teeth
- ☐ Rotated teeth
- ☐ Bridges or partial dentures
- ☐ Orthodontic braces
- ☐ Severe gum disease with bone loss, especially combined with any of the above

There are almost as many oddball brushes available as special dental problems requiring them. For example, interproximal brushes are designed to reach areas where a regular toothbrush, because of its size, does not have access, such as spaces created by bone loss between the teeth and around bridges and implants. When periodonal disease has set in and teeth have been lost or replaced, a standard toothbrush won't be sufficient to maintain your oral health. Your hygienist or dentist can recommend the interproximal brush that is best for your needs.

If you have a special dental problem and would like to know if there is a brush that will clean your teeth and gums better than the standard-size one you're using now, you should try an interproximal brush, a gingival crevice brush, an orthodontic brush, or a brush with bristles on the end. Butler makes all four of these brushes, and in my opinion they're the best of the lot. If you can't find them in stores you should ask your hygienist to order them for you. Remember, special problems require special solutions. Also keep in mind that the more efficient your dental tool is, the more time you'll save.

How many toothbrushes do you need? The number depends on the condition of your gums. If your gums are healthy and you have no bone loss you could get by with three: your regular brush, a hard-bristle brush for those special scrubbing times, and a hard-bristle brush to clean the toothbrushes. If you have periodontal disease with bone loss, you'll have to add periodontal or interproximal brushes that effectively deal with unique dental conditions. Your hygienist will tell you what you need.

There are many advantages to having at least two. First, you'll always have a spare if you lose the first one or if someone decides to use yours to clean the car's carburetor. Second, by having two brushes you can use one while the other is drying. I've also found it worthwhile to keep an extra in my traveling kit. I used to forget to put one in when I traveled and then I would have to buy a new one—this is one way of accumulating brushes, but I don't recommend it.

Keeping your brush clean In case you didn't know, the toothbrush is a very good germ incubator. The food particles and moisture that become trapped at the bottom of the bristles provide everything that germs need to reproduce rapidly . . . right on your very own brush. Research has shown that an unclean brush can contribute to dental disease by introducing germs from your brush into your mouth. This frustrates your hygiene program and can contribute to colds and sore throats. Studies have also shown that toothbrushes may contain more bacteria after they have sat for a time than immediately after you have brushed. So, you can see that an unclean brush will go against what you're trying to accomplish with oral hygiene, that is, to reduce the number of bacteria in your mouth. What this means is that you should sanitize (even boiling will not completely sterilize your brush) your brush after each brushing. Plus, you should never share your brush with anyone else because you don't want their germs, and they don't want yours. Of the two types of bristles, the natural fiber ones tend to breed more germs because they are more porous and attract and hold more water than the synthetic ones.

Here are my suggestions for keeping your brush as clean as possible.

☐ Rinse your brush thoroughly with hot water after each use, even when you use it without toothpaste.

☐ Let it drain by standing it on its handle in a glass or placing it in a toothbrush holder. Never let it lie flat with the bristles pointing to the sky.

☐ Alternate brushes so that they have a chance to dry out completely. Germs hate it when brushes dry out because they die when their environment is not moist enough.

☐ Use a hard-bristle brush to clean the bristles of your regular toothbrush every week, or as needed. This is easy to do, just like cleaning a hairbrush. While running your toothbrush under water, as hot as you can stand, scrub it thoroughly with the hard-bristle brush. When you've cleaned it, rinse it in hot water and hang it out to dry.

☐ Change brushes often. Some dentists recommend using a new brush every two weeks. If you have advanced periodontal disease or a depressed immune system some dentists say you should change your brushes more often. Those with infectious disease should change brushes at the onset of the disease and when the disease has subsided.

☐ Sanitizing devices and agents. There are several ways to sanitize your toothbrush. Purebrush uses ultraviolet light. It effectively reduces the germ count, is easy to use, and has a place to store toothbrushes. NuBrush uses an antibacterial agent to reduce the germ count.

How long will a toothbrush last? This is an intriguing question. The answer depends on how hard or soft the bristles are and how much the toothbrush is used. A soft brush, given the same amount of usage, will wear out sooner than a hard one. Used properly, the average toothbrush will wear out in three to six months. If yours lasts a year, which is about how long most people use a brush, it means one of three things. It's worn out and you're waiting too long to buy a new one. If it's still in good shape it means you haven't used it enough. Or, the bristles of your brush are too hard, even if the label says it's a medium or soft. The best criterion to use for replacing a brush is really simple. If you're diligently following your hygiene program, let the actual condition of the brush be your guide.

When it gets all gunked up or when the bristles start to flatten, it's time to replace the brush, no matter how long you've been using it. It's also a good idea to change to a new brush after each hygiene visit.

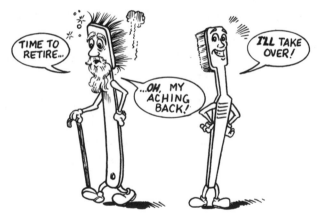

This is a perfect time to start fresh because you don't want to introduce bacteria found on your brush into your mouth after a good cleaning.

Electric Toothbrushes

Electric toothbrushes have been a valuable addition to toothbrush technology. There are a number of these on the market, and although they come in different sizes, shapes, and colors, they all have one thing in common: they rotate the bristles faster than any human hand can. I call them the lazy person's toothbrush. But whether they rotate four thousand times a minute or a thousand, go clockwise or counterclockwise, you still have to control them. This means you have to use them when you should and at the proper angle. If you find that you have not been able to solve your hygiene problem with a regular toothbrush, then give the electric toothbrush a try. Personally, I like the Panasonic Powerfloss the best. It's not just an electric toothbrush but an electric flosser as well. It has a case to store and protect the brushes, and it's ADA-approved.

Toothpaste

Oh boy! There now seem to be about as many brands of toothpaste as there are makes of cars. There are pastes, powders, and gels; whiteners and brighteners; fluoridated pastes, flavored ones, those that contain baking soda, and pastes for sensitive teeth. What to do? Oh, what to do? Well, I won't presume to tell you what to do, but I will give you the information you need to make your own choice.

Why pastes? Toothpaste was originally invented to clean the teeth of food debris and unsightly stains. When toothpaste was first marketed, very little was known about the cause of dental disease, but people did know enough to realize that it was more appealing to keep their teeth clean than to leave them dirty. The first toothpastes were either too abrasive, too acidic, toxic, yucky-tasting, or all of the above. From that humble beginning, toothpaste making has grown into a multibillion-dollar-a-year industry. One that markets its products with every conceivable come-on—from sex appeal to promises of decay and plaque reduction.

Over the years, government regulations have forced manufacturers of toothpastes to clean up their act and let consumers know what they're actually getting for their buck. These regulations have helped, but I do not believe that they have protected the consumer as much as they should. For example, do you know what toothpastes contain and why they're composed of these substances? Thought so. At any rate, I recommend that you *never* swallow your toothpaste, even if you do know what it contains.

Toothpaste categories All toothpastes fall into one of two categories. They are either therapeutic or cosmetic. Therapeutic toothpastes must contain ingredients, like fluoride, that have been shown to prevent or significantly reduce tooth decay and gingivitis. To be labeled "therapeutic" a toothpaste must be approved by the American Dental Association. If you are unsure about which product you should buy, and one is labeled "ADA accepted" but the other is not, select the one approved by the ADA.

The makers of cosmetic dentifrices (*dentifrice* refers to all kinds of tooth cleansers, from pastes and gels to powders) promote these products for their ability to make your teeth whiter and brighter. These products either bleach the tooth itself or remove stains through abrasion or acid etching. Some manufacturers may suggest that their toothpastes are both cosmetic and therapeutic, but unless they directly attack the disease process, manufacturers cannot claim that their products are therapeutic.

Toothpaste ingredients Although the ingredients, and their proportions, of many toothpastes are closely guarded secrets, most toothpastes (including therapeutic pastes) contain all or some of the following substances:

1. ABRADING, POLISHING, AND BLEACHING AGENTS   Abrading and polishing agents comprise as much as 50 percent of most dentifrices. The abrasive ingredient actually grinds off enamel and dentin, much like rough sandpaper abrades wood. The polishing agents are included to help smooth off the roughened areas, like using a fine sandpaper to smooth the roughness. The extent to which any dentifrice will abrade your teeth will depend on the following factors:

☐ Its abrasive index (which I'll explain in a moment)

☐ Its acidity

☐ The hardness of your tooth enamel

☐ The hardness of the toothbrush bristles

☐ The force with which you use your brush

☐ How long and how often you brush

Thus, you could use an abrasive toothpaste but not brush very hard or very often and therefore not wear away as much tooth as if you used a less abrasive paste, used hard bristles, brushed hard, and brushed often. Clear?

As you will see in the home care chapter (Chapter 5), abrading and polishing agents can be valuable if they are used correctly. But toothpastes that are highly acidic or abrasive—I call these toothpastes "glamour pastes"—can be double-edged swords if they are abused. Originally intended to remove dietary and other stains, such as those caused by coffee, tea, and tobacco, some of these pastes contain acids that are actually powerful enough to remove tooth enamel and dentin. This is especially true if you have soft teeth.

You may not know it, but although enamel is pretty hard and looks solid white, it is actually somewhat translucent. The dentin, the supportive tooth substance that lies directly underneath the enamel, is yellow in color. Hmmm, just what's he getting at? Just this: as the enamel wears away and gets thinner, the dentin shows through more and more. And because the dentin is yellow, guess what seems to be happening to your teeth? Yep, they'll appear to be yellowing. Although enamel can be intrinsically stained during its formation and varies in color, the truth is that, once it has formed, the enamel itself never actually becomes yellow, it just becomes thinner, pitted, or stained. If the enamel is intrinsically stained, or if it has been getting thinner, using a strong abrasive or etching agent defeats the whole purpose of the whiter-and-brighter promotion, doesn't it?

Many people are born with yellow-looking teeth. This could be the result of thinner, colored, or more translucent enamel or of dentin that is more yellow than normal. If you find yourself in this category, don't fall into the whitener paste trap. When you first use a whitener, you may think your teeth are getting whiter because the toothpaste removes the surface stains. If you only use such pastes periodically to remove dietary stains and then stop, you will be using them correctly. But if the continual search for those movie-star whites (most of which are capped, anyway) has led you to think that scrubbing and polishing your enamel away is the right way to go, you're barking up the wrong tree.

You have every right to want to look as good as you can, but there's a better way to whiten your teeth—without damaging them.

Bottom line, don't get sucked in by toothpastes that promise you unrealistic results. The good news is that the whiter-and-brighter toothpaste manufacturers seem to be getting the message, and some of these companies are cutting back on abrasive and acidic ingredients and are replacing them with bleaching agents, which makes these pastes less harmful to your enamel. But they still are not nearly as effective as having your teeth whitened and brightened at the dental office.

If you are dead set on using this kind of paste, I have a suggestion. First go to the RDH to get a good dose of hygiene therapy. She uses a paste containing pumice, one of the most powerful and safe abrasives. Believe me, once your teeth have been scraped and polished, they will be as white as they will ever be from brushing. They couldn't get any whiter if you brushed with an acidic or abrasive paste two hundred times a day. If they still are not as white as you would like, then ask your dentist if he thinks a professional bleaching will do the trick. (Bleaching is discussed in detail in Chapter 13.)

Abrasive and acidic pastes not only wear away the enamel; they can also erode and dull composite fillings and older plastic fillings. Also, soft teeth will be worn away faster than hard teeth by the same abrasive action.

THE ABRASIVE INDEX Thankfully, there is a measuring system that is used to monitor the abrasiveness of any substance. On the abrasive index, the lower the number, the less abrasive the material. As a rule, a substance with an abrasive index under 70 will not abrade fillings or enamel, or will do so very slowly; it will, however, wear away the dentin of an exposed root, because the root surface is much softer than enamel. Any substance that has an index ranging from 70 to 100 can begin to wear away soft enamel. Anything above 100 could wear most enamel. How fast an abrading substance will wear away enamel depends on its abrasive index, the hardness of your enamel, and how often you use the abrading substance. (In fact, the brush alone, without paste, is able to abrade the root surface.)

When choosing a dentifrice, it is valuable for you to know which abrasive has the highest abrasive index. So if you want control, read the labels.

If you run across an abrasive substance with which you are not familiar, your dentist or hygienist will be able to tell you its abrasive index. Remember, by itself, baking soda is a powerful abrasive. Even salt is somewhat abrasive.

The Most Common Abrasives	ABRASIVE INDEX
Zirconium silicate	Over 150
Pumice	Over 150
Calcium carbonate	Over 125
Anhydrous dicalcium phosphate	110 to 130
Calcium pyrophosphate	105
Insoluble sodium metaphosphate	100
Dihydrate dicalcium phosphate	25 to 75

2. BINDERS Binders, like sodium carboxymethylcellulose (one of those typical household words), are substances that keep together the liquid and solid parts of the toothpaste or gel. Some other commonly used binders are tragacanth, karaya gum, and gum arabic. These are natural substances from plants. Alginates from seaweed, gum carrageenan, xanthan gum, and cellulose derivatives are also popular binders. You can feel pretty good about all these substances.

3. ANTI-DRYING AGENTS (HUMECTANTS) Humectants are chemical compounds that help prevent the gel or paste from drying out when it contacts air. The three most commonly used are sorbitol (also used as a sweetener), glycerol, and propylene glycol. Humectants comprise a substantial part of the paste, about 25 percent.

4. DETERGENTS, OR FOAMING AGENTS Yep, many toothpastes have a soap ingredient to help cleanse and bubble away the bad guys. There's not much chance of these detergents removing the layers of plaque that have become firmly attached to the teeth, but they can have an effect on germs either by foaming them away like your laundry detergent does dirt or, in some cases, by killing them. Regular soap used to be common in toothpastes, but so many people complained about the bad taste that manufacturers stopped

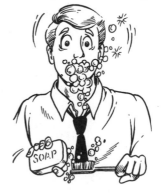

using it. Now most toothpastes contain a compound called sodium lauryl sulfate. I think it's also found in some shampoos. Although it too is a detergent, it's a more palatable one. Other common detergents are sodium coconut monoglyceride sulfonate, dioctyl sodium sulfosuccinate, and sodium N-lauroyl sarcosinate. This last one is believed to have some antibacterial actions. Detergents make up only about 3 percent of the toothpaste.

5. FLAVORING AGENTS Flavor is not necessary for a toothpaste to fulfill its purpose, but it is necessary if the toothpaste is going to sell. Flavoring agents can range from natural essential oils such as peppermint, wintergreen, glove, anise, and cinnamon to purely synthetic flavors with long-winded chemical names. Those in charge of marketing toothpastes have figured out that not everyone's taste buds are the same, and just as when people shop for cars, people like to have a choice. Free enterprise in action.

6. SWEETENERS Most dentifrices add a sweetener to go along with the flavoring agent. The good news is that I haven't found one brand of toothpaste that uses sugar as a sweetener, although I believe some of them used to. The most common sweetener is saccharin. If using saccharin is a personal dietary problem take the time to write the manufacturer of your favorite toothpaste to find out if they use it.

7. COLORING AGENTS Does anyone seriously think that teeth or germs care about the color of toothpaste? But we humans seem to care a great deal. So we get reds and blues and red-and-white candy cane twists. We also get FD&C yellow #5, FD&C yellow #20, FD&C green #3, and about twenty other FD&Cs. In my opinion, artificial coloring agents found in commercial toothpastes are unnecessary, but as long as you make sure you rinse well, are not allergic to them, and do not swallow the stuff, you should be fine. The choice is yours.

8. WATER Wow, we finally get to a pure and natural substance. Water makes up about 25 percent of your toothpaste.

9. PRESERVATIVES Back to the artificial. The most common preservative used in toothpaste is sodium benzoate. This compound is also used as a preservative in many foods. If you're concerned about preservatives check your toothpaste label. Ingesting a lot of

them may not be healthy. Most toothpastes use preservatives to control the possibility of germs feeding on some of the other, more natural compounds found in the ingredients. Get ready for this: among the preservatives used are formaldehyde, paraben, and dichlorophene.

10. ANTIPLAQUE AGENTS Fluoride and other chemicals, because of their ability to kill or inhibit germs, are often added to toothpastes. Whether or not you need this type of paste is up to you and your hygienist to decide. If you find you are unable to keep your teeth and gums healthy using a nonfluoridated toothpaste you should give a fluoridated one a try.

Natural pastes I recommend that you use natural toothpastes. Natural toothpastes are those that have no artificial ingredients. You're going to assimilate some of the compounds found in the toothpaste whether you absorb the ingredients through the tissues of the mouth or actually swallow them. I personally would rather ingest natural substances than artificial ones. And if you have children, you certainly don't want them getting any more chemicals than they are already ingesting and absorbing. I recommend Tom's of Maine.

If you feel it's in your best interest to use a natural toothpaste here are a couple of things to consider:

☐ Check the abrasive ingredient and then check the list on page 101 to find its rating on the abrasive index. Then decide whether this paste should be your regular one or saved for special use. Make sure that you use a highly abrasive paste for stain removal only or when you have missed a regular brushing or two.

☐ Look for one that tastes good. As I have said before, taste is unimportant as far as your teeth are concerned, but if you really don't like the taste it may prevent you from brushing as often as you should. This is especially true for children. Don't settle for a toothpaste that is natural but tastes lousy, and be sure to ask your child's opinion. Please, as a special favor to me, skip the "I like it so you should too" or "It's the cheapest" or "We have to use it up first" rationales.

Toothpastes by themselves will never cure or prevent dental disease whether they are standard or natural. After all, you could chew on toothpaste twenty times a day, but if you never put it on a brush and start scrubbing it would do very little to prevent dental disease.

What about the container? Most toothpaste tubes are lined with an inert substance so that the chemicals in the paste will not react with the lining of the tube and create some weird, harmful compound. Some tubes are lined with aluminum, and most scientists agree that too much aluminum is not healthy. Whenever possible, buy toothpastes that come in plastic containers. I am no great lover of plastics, but it's the safe alternative to avoid chemical interactions, particularly lead contamination since lead is sometimes used to seal the seams of metal containers.

Sensitivity to toothpastes Some people are sensitive to various ingredients found in toothpastes. Their reactions range from mild irritation and burning sensations to inflammation of the mucous membrane, swelling, and even ulcerations of the oral membranes (the skin found in the mouth). These effects are even more pronounced if a person already has open sores or inflamed or infected gums.

The most common irritants found in toothpaste are detergents and essential oils, like clove or peppermint. Pay attention to the sensations in your mouth when you're brushing and soon after. If you notice any symptoms, try brushing a few days without paste and see if they disappear. If you have a sensitive mouth or are susceptible to cold sores or herpes, the irritants found in pastes could make your condition worse and be a contributing factor to its initiation. If you think your paste might be a contributing factor try changing to a blander toothpaste, one that contains no detergents and no essential oils. If you make the change and the symptoms go away, the culprit could very well be in the paste. If irritation persists keep changing brands, but be sure to speak with your dentist or hygienist about this, because the cause may be something more serious than an allergy to an ingredient found in your toothpaste.

Tooth powders Most tooth powders seem to be going the way of the buffalo: they're still around, but not the way they used to be. You may be sold on them, and if they work for you then keep on using them. Just be sure to check your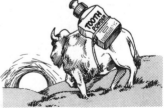

tooth powder's abrasiveness. One natural tooth powder that is becoming popular now is Eco-dent, made by Mer-flu-an. It's not only a good way to clean your teeth but has been proven effective in re-mineralizing the enamel. Look for it at your health food store.

Pastes for Special Problems

There are toothpastes that are specifically formulated to treat sensitive teeth—teeth that are sensitive to the normal ranges of hot and cold food and drinks, air temperature, brushing, acidic foods like lemons, or basic substances like baking soda. When teeth are sensitive like this, what's happening is that some of the nerve endings are being exposed to the outside environment. But unless you are aware of the specific *cause* of your sensitivity, you probably will be wasting your money buying toothpastes that are supposed to reduce it. Tooth sensitivity can be caused by new fillings, decay, fractures, or exposed root surfaces. None of these pastes will permanently alleviate sensitivity caused by new fillings, and they may only temporarily relieve sensitivity caused by decay and fractures and may even irritate a decayed area. This type of toothpaste does have value, though, when used temporarily to treat root sensitivity. If your sensitivity is due to exposed root surfaces, you may be using an overly abrasive dentifrice that is wearing away the mineral deposits that form inside and over the dentin tubules. These microscopic tubules contain fluid and connect the outside of the dentin to the pulp's nerve. Even though the tubules themselves don't contain actual nerve endings they, in effect, act as nerve endings, because they transmit the external irritant (be it heat, cold, or chemical) to the nerve. If abrasion continues, the minerals deposited by your saliva and the secondary dentin that is deposited in the outer portion of the tubules will not be able to seal the tubules and the sensitivity will continue. If you stop abrading the dentin, these tubules will seal themselves and the sensitivity should stop. It is truly amazing what the body can do.

Unfortunately, many patients use paste for sensitive teeth as they would aspirin, to help relieve the symptoms, and often avoid permanent long-term treatment when the pain subsides. But it is the cause that needs to be addressed, not just the symptoms. When the cause has been eliminated (you have repaired the decay, cured the gum disease, are brushing in the right way, have stopped sucking on lemons, etc.), the sensitivity should go away on its own within two weeks. As long as you are working with the dentist to treat the real cause of the sensitivity, I see no reason not to use these antisensitivity toothpastes to help relieve the symptoms. I believe the best over-the-counter toothpaste for sensitive teeth is Protect. But remember, if you have sensitivity, are using this kind of paste, and are not seeing a dentist, you could be masking the symptoms of a more serious problem.

Baking Soda

The best use of baking soda is for baking and for scouring pots and pans. However, it does have a use in your oral hygiene program, under controlled conditions. Pure baking soda is a valuable cleansing aid and can be used when you have been unable to brush for a day or more and as a once-a-week tooth scrub. Some toothpastes have baking soda in them, giving you that abrasive quality in a more palatable form. For the every-so-often super scrub, however, use it straight. But remember, it is a highly abrasive substance and you should use it with discretion. Another caution: baking soda contains sodium that can be assimilated through the permeable oral membranes or even swallowed during brushing and rinsing. If you're on a low-sodium diet I do not recommend that you use baking soda without approval from your doctor.

Baking soda also has value because it neutralizes the acid produced by bacteria. Some people actually use baking soda as a mouthwash, and if you don't have a dietary problem with sodium this is an excellent and inexpensive way not only to neutralize oral acids but to freshen breath. Always remember to rinse and gargle well after using baking soda. It will reduce the amount of sodium you absorb.

Salt

Salt has value as an antibacterial agent when used to treat gum disease, especially when used with an oral irrigation device. But once your gums have healed, I suggest that you only use it occasionally, if at all. Because the relationship between salt and heart attacks is too conclusive to be denied, there is no reason to add more sodium to your system by overusing it in your oral hygiene program. You can always use hydrogen peroxide or other antibacterial agents. Remember, only use something that gives results and causes no harm.

Dental Floss

If the toothbrush is king, floss is the queen. If you have gum disease or if you've had any bone loss, floss is an absolute must for a successful hygiene program. This magical material is used to clean and polish between the teeth and under dental appliances. If used daily it can prevent plaque from forming in these areas and can remove food wedged between the teeth that a toothbrush cannot budge. But don't ever think that you can avoid a visit to the hygienist by using floss on calculus: floss will never remove calculus. However, floss is truly one of the best preventive tools you can use. It is versatile, easy to carry, and, once you learn how, easy to use.

There are three main kinds of floss—waxed, unwaxed, and the newest kind, coated with silicone. There are also flosses that are impregnated with baking soda and fluoride. Floss is made in different thicknesses and widths. Your choice of floss is personal, practical, and functional. There are more than twenty different brands, so discovering the best type for you may end up being a trial-and-error process. Take a short-cut and ask your hygienist or dentist which kind of floss is most appropriate for your particular situation. See pages 126–31 for how to floss. If you have any trouble learning, ask them for guidance.

Waxed versus unwaxed I believe waxed floss is easier to use. It doesn't fray as easily and seems to slide between the contacts of the teeth better than does unwaxed floss. Because it doesn't fray so easily, it works better in areas where you have fillings. Some dentists and hygienists prefer unwaxed floss; they say it attacks plaque better than waxed floss because the wax coating interferes with the effectiveness of the floss on the plaque. Why not try them both? Then use the type with which you feel most comfortable.

Regular floss This is the most common kind of floss. It's thinner than dental tape, and most people feel it is easier to use, including me. In most cases it will do the job for you. Some brands are thinner than others and thus slide more easily through tight contacts.

Dental tape   This is a wider, and usually thicker, form of floss. It is most effective when you've had bone loss and gum recession. It is more effective than regular floss when there's a lot of root surface to clean and polish. I've had patients who swear by dental tape.

There are many brands of dental floss on the market, but my personal choice is Butler's G • U • M dental floss. They make every type: regular, tape, fine, shred-resistant, and flavored. Regardless of which brand you buy, you must use it, and use it correctly, to get results.

Floss holders   There are a number of handy little dental gadgets on the market that look like miniature slingshots. These are called "floss holders." Basically, they hold the floss tightly between two plastic arms attached to a handle. The one I recommend to my patients is called the FlossMate, made by Butler. When you are first developing your flossing technique, holders may seem easier to use, but I like the control I have when I use my fingers. If you just can't master the manual use of floss, try a holder. However, many patients and hygienists have told me that floss holders are harder to control when you're trying to floss all areas of the root surface, especially if there has been bone loss. There is a tendency to slam the floss straight down into the gum between the teeth. This can cause injury to the gum tissue. It may seem difficult to learn how use floss manually, but the results will be worth the effort.

Floss threaders   Bridges require a special tool to reach the areas under the bridge and keep these areas free of plaque and food debris. Yep, plaque and calculus can even form on artificial teeth. While there are a number of bridge threaders, the product I like best is Butler's Eez-Thru floss threader. The floss threader has a large loop and can be easily threaded under bridges and orthodontic appliances.

Mouthwash

The value of mouthwash goes beyond its use as a fighter of bad breath. They are effective in the treatment of gingivitis. There are many brands of mouthwashes on the market, and although they have differing formulas, colors, and tastes, they all have one thing in common—they reduce the number of germs found in your mouth. A mouthwash's effectiveness will depend on how it's delivered to your gums and how often you use it. Both rinsing and delivering the mouthwash through a water irrigation device will produce good results: reduced bleeding, reduced gingivitis, and reduced plaque formation. But the best results are achieved when the mouthwash is used twice a day (after you brush and floss) with a water irrigation device. You can use the mouthwash at full strength, but a solution of equal parts water and mouthwash is also very effective and is less expensive. The water irrigation device is more effective because it delivers the germ-fighting ingredients to the gingival crevice, or pocket.

Rinsing with mouthwash after brushing and flossing is about 50 percent as effective as irrigating with it. Use mouthwash at full strength when rinsing, and be sure to forcefully suck the solution between your teeth. If you rinse well with water before you use the mouthwash it will be more effective. You should include mouthwash in your hygiene program until your hygienist gives you a clean bill of health. After your gums have healed you should be able to keep them healthy without mouthwash, and its further use will be up to you. If you do continue using a mouthwash in a preventive way the two best times are after your final brushing of the day and following the ingestion of anything that contains sugar (if you are unable brush). There are two groups of mouthwash, prescription and over-the-counter.

Prescription mouthwashes Peridex is the most common prescription mouthwash. The active ingredient is called chlorhexidine. Studies have shown it to be more effective at reducing plaque and gingivitis than over-the-counter mouthwashes. It is also approved by the Food and Drug Administration and the ADA. But, like all drugs, it is not without its side effects. Prolonged use can cause tooth stains, increased supragingival calculus formation, and gum irritation in children. Like most drugs, its effect on pregnant and nursing mothers is inconclusive. Always consider the potentially harmful side effects before using any prescription drug. Its effectiveness and safety with children under eighteen has not yet been established. It also contains alcohol.

Peridex has its place in treating gingivitis and reducing plaque, but unless your dentist feels it is absolutely necessary, I would try over-the-counter mouthwashes first. If they don't get results, Peridex might. Remember that without the willingness to use your brush, floss, oral irrigator, and hygienist to fight this disease, mouth-wash will be like attempting to put out a fire with a squirt gun.

Over-the-counter mouthwashes Although the active ingre-dients used in these mouthwashes vary, they all claim to do the same thing. Of all the mouthwashes available, both standard and natural, I recommend Mer-flu-an. It's free of alcohol and contains no artificial ingredients. Also, it's concentrated and one bottle makes a gallon of mouthwash.

A number of mouthwashes contain fluoride. Stannous fluo-ride has been approved by the ADA for its antidecay properties, and though some studies have shown that fluoride reduces plaque, its ability to help heal gingivitis is questionable. Many commercial mouthwashes also contain alcohol and salt. Be sure to read the la-bels, and if either of these substances is a health concern switch to a mouthwash that fills your needs.

Because mouthwash reduces the mouth's salivary and airborne germ count, many dentists and hygienists have their patients rinse with mouthwash before and after hygiene therapy and dental re-pair. If this is not the standard policy in your dentist's office, ask them if you can rinse before they begin and after they finish. By kill-ing germs, the mouthwash can promote the healing process.

Gum

What—gum is a dental tool? Yep, and an effective one, at that. Within minutes after eating a meal containing sugar, the acid level of the mouth rises, and the acid concentration can remain high for many hours if not removed or neutralized. Gum chewing promotes the flow of saliva, and as you know, a healthy saliva flow can help neutralize the acid produced by bacteria—that makes it a decay fighter and an effective between-meal brushing dental tool, espe-cially after eating anything that contains sugar. Rinsing vigorously with water before you chew makes the gum even more effective. Chew for at least twenty minutes. Do not chew gum that contains sugar, because the saliva will have to neutralize the sugar in the gum as well as the sugar in the food you just ate. Of the sugarless gums available, Tart-X Sugar Free Tartar Control Gum is the best natural chewing gum I've found. It's not only a chewing gum that stimu-lates saliva flow, but it also contains microfibers that act as miniature brushes to clean the teeth and massage the gums. You can find it at some health food stores, or you can order it by calling 800-248-0107. Peelu also makes a good natural chewing gum.

Gum has an additional benefit: chewing it exercises the jaw muscles, and that can help relieve the tension many people store there. But if you have TMJ problems, gum chewing isn't recommended.

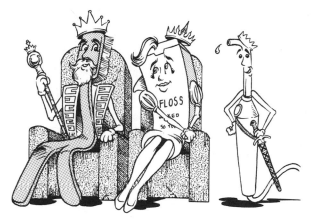

Water Irrigation Devices

If the toothbrush is king, and floss is queen, then the water irrigating device is the crown prince. If you have advanced gum disease and bone loss, or if you can't seem to keep your gums healthy using the brush and floss, this device could make the difference between losing and keeping your teeth. Its value is not just in treating gum disease but also in preventing it. So don't wait until you have gum disease to start using one. It is truly a wonderful invention and I use it regularly.

The basic concept behind the water irrigator is to shoot a pulsating stream of water out of a nozzle. The most efficient devices have controls that let you regulate the amount of pressure they deliver. When used in the right way, at the right time, and directed to the right areas, this little machine removes food debris and germs, dislodges newly forming plaque, massages the gums, and delivers antibacterial agents to areas that other dental aids never reach. These devices, wonderful as they are, will never replace the brush or floss—but they sure can help both of them.

Types of irrigating devices Many brands and types of oral irrigators are available. Most are electrically powered, but there are a few that have a universal attachment that lets you hook them up to a water faucet. This is fine if you have both hot and cold water coming out of one faucet, but there are still many sinks that have hot water coming out of one faucet and cold out of the other, which means you cannot control the water temperature. If this is your situation get an electric irrigator because you absolutely must be able to adjust the temperature of the water to your body temperature. The type that hooks up to a faucet is great for people without electricity.

Having tried most of these devices I feel that the Water Pik Oral Irrigator is the best. Water Pik makes a wide selection, including a smaller version for traveling, and a new tip that reaches further into the gum's pocket.

Toothpicks: Picking a Pick

Toothpicks come in great variety, ranging from the slender pieces of wood we all know to many kinds of plastic and rubber ones. All are effective interdental stimulators, and used correctly, any toothpick can provide a lot of support for your oral hygiene efforts. The critical thing is to fully understand what a pick can and cannot do so that you won't misuse this important tool. Toothpicks *can* be abused. During one three-year period, from 1979 to 1982, there were over twenty-four thousand toothpick-related injuries. Most of these injuries were to the eyes and ears of children. The most serious injuries resulted when toothpicks were swallowed. Be careful.

Stim-U-Dent This is one of the handiest and most effective of the interdental stimulators. It is easy to use and the choice of many dental professionals. It is also easy to find—most drugstores and dental departments of supermarkets carry them.

Wooden toothpicks These come in different sizes and shapes. I prefer the triangular ones, but any of them will work if used correctly. Hand-held toothpicks do not give you access to the spaces between and around the back teeth as efficiently as toothpicks with handles.

Plastic toothpicks Since these are available in many sizes and shapes, you should ask your hygienist which one is best for you. These have handles that give you better control.

Rubber toothpicks These are nice because of their flexibility. And because they don't have a sharp, hard point, you're less likely to harm the gum tissue if you accidentally poke yourself.

Homemade toothpicks In a pinch, you can use carved pieces of wood, small twigs, and just about anything else that is clean and reaches the areas you want to pick. Feel free to be creative. Don't use a sharp point and, before using, fray the end by chewing on it.

Toothpick holders These are great. Their unique handles are designed to hold a wooden toothpick. They give better control and greater access to the gums, are easy to use, and can make a big difference in your oral hygiene program. The one I like the best is called the Perio Aid, made by the Marquis Dental Manufacturing Company. This brand comes in different styles and sizes, and the picks are packaged in a handy case that holds extra toothpicks. You should be able to find them at the drugstore, but many dental offices either sell them or give them away. Your hygienist may have a style she likes best, so be sure to ask her about them and have her show you where and how to use them.

Disclosing Agents

Disclosing agents are colored tablets or liquids containing a vegetable dye. When the dye reaches the teeth, it stains the food debris and plaque a reddish or purple color. It will not stain the teeth themselves.

Just remember, the color doesn't wear off immediately, so you might not want to use a disclosing agent before going out on a date. It can also stain your clothes and should not be swallowed. Always use it according to the directions. Butler makes disclosing agents in both tablet and liquid form, and you can find them at any drugstore or at your dentist's.

SOMETHING TO THINK ABOUT

It is one thing to know about available preventive tools and another to know how, when, and where to use them. There is no free lunch. Your choice is between keeping your teeth for the rest of your life or losing them. None of these tools have brains, legs, or arms. Without you, they can do nothing for your teeth and gums, so if you don't use them, you will lose them . . . not your tools, your teeth. The next chapter tells you how to put your tools to work.

The Tooth Fitness Digest (see Appendix) will constantly give you updates on the latest and greatest dental aids, but if you find that you still have questions about which ones would be best for you, be sure to ask your hygienist.

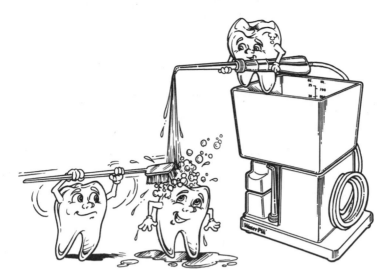

Chapter 5

Your Personal
Home Care Program

Well, we've covered a lot of ground together. Now you understand the cause of tooth decay and gum disease. You also know how to perform a self-examination and which tools you need to fight these diseases. But acquiring knowledge is not enough. You must turn that knowledge into action. If you're ready to do that, this is the chapter that will show you how.

When you have integrated what you learn in this chapter with the instructions and guidance your hygienist and dentist provide, you will have an oral hygiene program that is customized to your mouth. However, understand that no matter how well your hygiene program is designed, you must also be willing to include all of the following actions as part of your total preventive program:

☐ Have existing tooth and gum disease treated and repaired. Remember, you must first get rid of the disease before you can prevent its return.

☐ Do as much as you can to change your diet from a disease-promoting one to a disease-preventing one.

□ Resolve to brush, irrigate, floss, pick, or perform any combination of these activities immediately after eating any refined or processed foods.

□ Periodically do a self-examination.

□ Follow the hygiene recall schedule established by your hygienist.

ALL ABOUT BRUSHING

Let's begin with brushing, since brushing is the most basic home care procedure. The purpose of brushing your teeth is to accomplish two basic things:

1. To rid your mouth of all food and plaque from your mouth

2. To massage your gums

When to Brush

Any time is a good time to brush, but some times are better times than others. The most crucial times are after eating and in the morning. Brush immediately after eating, especially if the meal or snack contained processed food and refined sugar. By "immediately," I mean as soon as possible, but absolutely within four to six hours after any meal. The damage caused by food left in your mouth is directly proportional to how long it is left there.

Brushing in the morning is vital, even if you don't eat breakfast. You need to break up plaque that formed during the night. Plaque actually forms more rapidly during sleep than during waking hours, because it doesn't require food to attach its gooey self to your teeth and because most of your body's natural plaque fighters—your tongue, lips, and saliva—are not nearly so active at night. Even if your bedtime brushing removes all available germ food, the remaining plaque-forming germs continue to do their thing. Therefore, the morning brushing is critical, even if you don't eat. If you do eat breakfast you can accomplish two goals with a single brushing by brushing after you eat. Otherwise, brush as soon as possible.

Finally, it's a good idea to brush before going to bed, even if you brushed after your last meal, in order break up the plaque that has formed since then. Even if you've skipped meals or are fasting, never let more than eight hours go by without putting a brush to your teeth. If you have advanced periodontitis your RDH may have you brush more often.

How to Hold the Brush

There is no one way to hold a toothbrush. The best way is the way that works best for you. You could hold it with your toes, as long as you get the job done. You'll find that whichever grip you use, you will have to shift the position of your thumb on the brush to comfortably reach every part of your teeth and gums, especially the inside surfaces. It is often easier to change your grip than to rotate your arm and your wrist. Experiment and see what I mean. When you show your hygienist your brushing technique, she'll see if your present grip allows you to effectively reach all the brushing areas.

Putting on the Paste

Add enough paste to cover about a third of the bristles. Run body-temperature water over the brush and paste for a few seconds to equalize the temperatures of brush, paste, and your teeth. I suggest that you get into the habit of doing this, especially if you have bone loss and/or teeth that are sensitive to cold. If you use a tooth powder, run warm water over the brush before you add enough powder to lightly cover the bristles. Before you begin brushing, rinse and gargle with water. This will make the brushing more effective.

How Much Time to Spend

The only way to find out how much time you need to spend on your hygiene program is to follow the guidelines suggested in this book and by your hygienist. Don't be concerned if someone else needs more or less time than you do. You're not worried about saving their teeth, just yours. Look at it this way: what's important is not how much time you have to spend saving your teeth, but how much time you *save* by taking care of them. It takes much more time to treat dental disease than it will ever take to prevent it.

The amount of time you put in to keep each area of your mouth healthy is determined by how much disease you have now or have had in the past. For example, an area that's in the early stages of gingivitis will require less time and attention than an area with advanced periodontitis. Also, as you will discover, certain areas are more susceptible to decay and gum disease than others. These areas will always require more care.

The results of your hygiene efforts will determine your total time expenditure. Thus, if you start out spending four minutes a day (no cheating!) and are unable to maintain healthy teeth and gums, you'll have to increase your time to six minutes, seven, or maybe more. On the other hand, if you've been spending ten minutes a day and each checkup proves that your mouth is in great shape, you can reduce the time until you reach a happy balance. There really is no need to spend more time on dental care than you need.

YOUR BRUSHING PATTERN

Most people have a haphazard brushing technique, if they have one at all. Usually the brushing process starts at the front teeth and ends up somewhere in the back. There seems to be no rhyme or reason to their brushing, and in most cases, the front teeth get the most attention. Areas that need the most work are often missed altogether. I bet you can't tell me how you brushed the last time you brushed—where you began and ended. Thought so. Well, establishing a pattern is one of the little known, but very important, parts of a good hygiene program. You have three guides to help you do this. The first is your hygienist. She'll tell you which areas need the most work and how well you're doing. The second is the results of your self-examination. The third, if you have periodontitis, is your individualized pocket depth chart—this gives you a road map that directs you to the problem areas.

Where to Brush

Everyone knows you should brush your teeth, but brushing your teeth is only half the battle. Gums need to be brushed as much as teeth do. Even though plaque forms only on the teeth, the gums need the stimulation that brushing, flossing, and water irrigation provide. This massaging action stimulates blood circulation and toughens the gums, in the same way that calluses form on hands and feet to protect them. So, when you think "teeth," think "gums" too.

Every part of every tooth must be brushed, especially the gingival sulcus and the gums down to one-third of an inch below the gum line. Think of the area to be brushed as consisting of four parts:

1. Inside surfaces of the teeth and gums

2. Outside surfaces of the teeth and gums

3. Back side of the last teeth and gums

4. Chewing surfaces of all teeth

Following the Pattern

I want you to pick one side of your mouth to begin brushing, then always start from this point. Let's start with the upper right side. (Lefties may want to start on the left side.) If this starting point is new to you, your movements may feel awkward at first. If you get a little frustrated, hang in there. Establishing a set starting and finishing point has nothing to do with brushing technique per se, but it does guarantee that you will cover all the bases, every single time.

It is very important that you always follow the sequence I've outlined in this chapter because it will ensure that you first brush the areas that normally get the least attention. The insides of your teeth and gums and the outsides of the back teeth are where the highest incidence of gum disease occurs. You don't want to spend time on the less vulnerable areas and run out of gas before you get to the problem areas. If you need a reminder, stick a Post-it on your mirror.

While you read through the following directions, pretend your index finger is a toothbrush and go through the motions.

☐ Inside surfaces: Beginning your new brushing pattern with the last tooth on the upper right side, move around the insides of the upper teeth to the last tooth on the upper left side. Move your finger down to the inside of the last tooth on the lower left side, and then around to the last tooth on the lower right side.

☐ Outside surfaces: Next, put your finger on the last tooth on the upper right side and "brush" along the outsides of the upper teeth to the last tooth on the upper left side. Drop down to the outside of the last tooth on the lower left side. Move your finger around the outsides of the lower teeth, and finish on the last tooth on the lower right side.

☐ Back surfaces of last teeth: Begin with the back of the last upper right tooth, then move to the upper left, then down to the lower left, and finally to the back of the last tooth on the lower right side. I think you get the picture. Always start and end on the same side, and if you space out somewhere in between you'll always know where you've been and where you're going. (Ah, if only life were so simple.)

☐ Chewing surfaces: Finally, you get to "brush" the chewing surfaces. Begin on the top of the last tooth on the upper right side, and "brush" all the chewing surfaces of the upper teeth until you reach last tooth on the upper left side. Let gravity direct your finger down to the chewing surface of the last tooth on your lower left side. Continue scrubbing the tops of your bottom teeth all the way around your jaw to the last tooth on the lower right side. I suggest you do the tops last; do the other, harder-to-reach areas first, before you run out of energy or get bored.

The number of times you repeat the pattern will vary depending on the condition of your gums, so it might end up being four times or ten times.

DOWN TO BUSINESS: HOW TO BRUSH

Now that you know why, where, when, and how much time to spend, you need to know how. Each of the four parts of your mouth must be brushed in a slightly different way. I know you'll be practicing diligently at home with your mirror as your guide, but it will still be necessary to have your hygienist watch you run through your brushing technique. She'll be like the movie director for your own oral hygiene motion picture. She'll fine-tune your newly acquired brushing technique to fit your mouth. Remember, different strokes for different folks. Here's how you brush each area.

Inside Surfaces of the Back Teeth and Gums

Hold the brush firmly against the gums at a forty-five-degree angle. Then move the brush from the gums to the teeth. As you do this, keeping pressure against the teeth and gums, rotate your wrist until the brush reaches the point where the gum meets the teeth, the gum line. Once there, gently direct the bristles into the groove, or gingival crevice, between the teeth and the gum. While continuing to exert gentle, but firm, pressure, vibrate the bristles in a small

circular motion. This will
also force the bristles into
the spaces between the
teeth. The gingival crev-
ice is the most critical
area. Pause here and make
sure that you spend the extra time to clean and massage this area thoroughly.

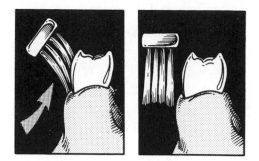

When you have taken care of the crevice, continue across the
rest of the tooth surface, increasing the pressure of the brush. With
an average-size brush, the bristles will effectively cover about two teeth

and the gums around them.
As you move the brush to
each new position, overlap
the last area you brushed
to avoid missing any area.

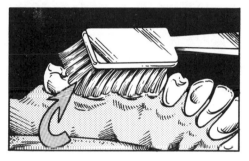

Never brush the teeth
from side to side. Over
time, brushing with a side-
to-side motion, especially if
you use abrasive toothpastes, can separate the gum from the tooth
and eventually wear a groove in the area of the root that is normally
protected by the gum.

Because the inside surfaces of your teeth are usually not given
as much attention as the outside surfaces, be sure to spend extra
time brushing them. Chances are good that if you check the condition of your gums around the insides of the back teeth, you will find
that they show signs of disease.

Inside Surfaces of the Front Teeth and Gums

These are the most difficult areas to reach with the brush. The
curvature of the inside of the front teeth makes it nearly impossible
to use the same technique on these teeth as you use for the rest of
your teeth. Reaching these areas is even more difficult for young
children and for people with small dental arches when the toothbrush is too large. Also, the fact that the mandibular salivary glands

lie directly below the lower front teeth makes this a potential trouble spot; most people tend to form a lot of calculus here.

So, after you've finished brushing the inside surfaces of the upper back teeth and you've reached the cuspid, what you'll need to do in order to reach the insides of the front teeth is to change the

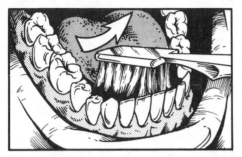

position of the brush. Use the drawing as a guide and angle the brush so that the tip of it is facing toward the back of the throat. Use the bristles that are closest to your hand to brush this area, both upper and lower. If you have any trouble keeping these areas clean and healthy you might have to switch to a children's brush.

Outside Surfaces of All Teeth

Use the same position and technique as you did with the inside surfaces of the back teeth and gums. Your toothbrush should be able to cover two teeth at once, but the key to the success of any brushing technique is not only how you brush but how much time

DR. TOM'S TIPS

You may be one of the many people who have trouble reaching the outsides of the last two upper teeth, on both sides, when your mouth is wide open. This happens because your lower jaw slides forward and literally pushes the brush out of the way when you open your mouth as far as you can, especially if you have a small mouth and use a big brush. To solve this problem, put the brush in your mouth, lay the brush flat against your upper back teeth in the position in which you would begin your brushing, and then close your mouth until the teeth are about one-half inch apart. Don't bite the brush. You will find you now have easy access to what was once a hard-to-reach area. Try it both ways and experience what I mean.

you spend in each area. When you and your hygienist have determined which teeth need the most attention you must give those areas extra time.

Back Surfaces of the Last Teeth

Place the brush in the position shown in the illustration below
and move it from left to
right in short strokes. The
size of most brushes makes
this movement a little
awkward and you need to
move the brush around to
clean both the tooth and
the gum. As when brush-
ing any area of your mouth,

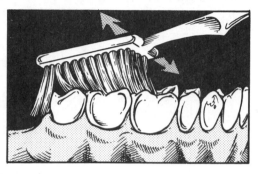

you have to take the trial-and-error path to discover the best approach. The backs of the last teeth are one of the most overlooked areas; so don't forget to hit these spots.

Chewing Surfaces

The developmental grooves of the back teeth run in all directions. If you are going to clean these grooves you will need to move the brush in all the directions in which the grooves run. Although it is not always possible to completely clean these grooves, a firm back-and-forth shimmy will clean them efficiently. Even if all the chewing surfaces have been restored with amalgam or composite fillings, it is still important to brush them because these fillings can break down or wear away where they meet the tooth. These mar-

gins are perfect breeding
grounds for germs and
ideal bases for plaque formation. Likewise, if you
have full crowns on your
back teeth you should still
brush the chewing por-
tion, because plaque can
form in the grooves and

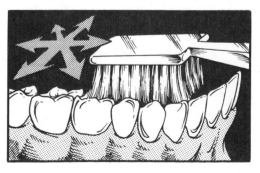

margins of a crown. Although this does not cause decay, the presence of plaque always means an increase in the germ population . . . and you know that's not good.

DRY BRUSHING

A growing number of dentists and hygienists are promoting dry brushing. The philosophy behind this technique is that dry bristles are more effective at dislodging plaque because neither toothpaste nor water comes between the bristle and the plaque. To dry brush, you do not have to change your brushing pattern or technique, and the only thing you do differently, aside from not adding paste or water, is to frequently wipe your saliva from the bristles with a cloth or tissue.

Combining dry and wet brushing negates the most undesirable aspect of each: the barrier created by paste and the unpalatable sensation (to me, anyway) of brushing dry. I suggest that you try a modified form of dry brushing in the morning. You wet the brush but do not use toothpaste—that is, if you brushed with paste the night before. I don't recommend dry brushing of any kind if you have gone more than twelve hours without brushing with paste. You need the more abrasive action of toothpaste to help dislodge plaque that has had extra time to adhere to the tooth.

At night, I suggest that you first apply toothpaste to the brush, then brush with it until you have completed a few full cycles around the teeth. That will take care of the cleaning and polishing of the teeth. When you've done that, rinse away the paste from the brush and your mouth and proceed with wet brushing. Most patients who have followed this procedure say it is easier to brush longer without the paste foaming up, and I agree.

WHICH TECHNIQUE SHOULD YOU USE?

There are many other brushing techniques besides the one I suggest, all variations on the same theme. And all of them require that you religiously follow their instructions. My brushing technique is not the only one that will work for you, but if you do it consistently you will establish an effective brushing routine. If your hygienist feels that your situation requires a modification of my technique, or even a totally different technique, for reasons she can explain to you, then take her advice and adjust your technique until your brushing generates the results you seek.

Remember, if you've had bone loss the brush alone will not be enough to keep your teeth and gums healthy. In these areas you need to use floss, a water irrigation device, mouthwashes, special brushes, and various kinds of interdental stimulators. The function of the toothbrush is unlike that of the other two main preventive tools—floss and water irrigation devices. Likewise, floss's function is unique, and neither can do what the water irrigation device does. Using a variety of preventive tools is like using a saw, a hammer, and a screwdriver in the right situation. You would never hammer a nail with a screwdriver . . . at least I hope not.

ABOUT FLOSSING

If you've never had gum disease; if you have perfect dental restorations, no bad contacts, a healthy diet; if you understand all the hows, whys, and whens of oral hygiene and are faithful to your hygiene program—you may never need to floss. Only a few percent of the population fall into this category, and if you're reading this book, I don't think you do.

Flossing removes food, breaks up plaque formations, cleans the teeth, and massages the gums—but does so only in the areas the floss can reach. For example, you can't floss the outsides or insides of your teeth, only the sides. The drawing shows where the floss and the brush clean. The shaded areas between the teeth, from 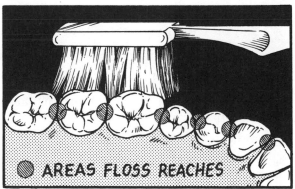 the top of the teeth down to the gums, are the only areas the floss can effectively reach. All other parts of the teeth and gums belong to the brush and the water irrigator. So now you can see why you need to do both—brush and floss.

You can floss anytime, but if you are brushing and flossing, floss after you brush.

HOW TO FLOSS

Understand, it is more difficult to read about how to floss from a book than it is to actually floss. Over the years I've seen about twenty different descriptions of how to floss, even though they all described the same procedure. Learning to floss correctly is no more difficult than learning to do it the wrong way, but only the correct method will get results. It may seem difficult and feel awkward in the beginning, but if you think your teeth are worth saving you won't give up until you get the technique down pat. With practice, and guidance from the hygienist, you'll soon be able to floss and think about something else at the same time.

The following description is for right-handed people, so if you're a lefty you'll have to make adjustments. Even if you already feel comfortable about your flossing method, stay tuned to make sure you're flossing correctly.

Part 1: Positions and Patterns

The first part of this section explains how to hold the floss and describes an effective flossing pattern. As with brushing, always start flossing on the same side. I always begin on the upper right side no matter which dental tool I am using, so I always have a reference point. So, start on either the upper right or upper left side, then move around to the opposite side, drop down to the lower jaw, and move around to finish on the side where you started.

1. Start with about eighteen inches of dental floss. If you find that you need more or less floss, be my guest.

2. Wrap the floss three or four times around the middle finger of your right hand at the level of the joint closest to your finger-nail. Do the same for the middle finger of the left hand. See figure 1.

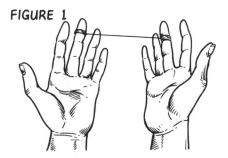

FIGURE 1

3. Adjust the floss so that there are about one to one and one-half inches of floss between your two fingers.

Flossing the upper jaw   Use one position for the right side and a slight variation of it for the left side.

UPPER RIGHT SIDE

1. Move the floss over the soft part of your right thumb, and use your index finger to hold the floss in place. Now, place the floss over the pad of your left index finger. See figure 2. (Thank goodness for artists.)

FIGURE 2

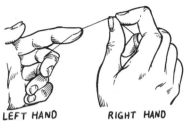

LEFT HAND   RIGHT HAND

2. Slowly move your hands apart until the floss is tightly stretched.

3. Place the index finger of your left hand in your mouth. Flossing will only work if your right finger and thumb are kept outside the teeth.

4. In order to practice, try this technique on your front teeth, where it is easiest, and when you feel confident, start with the last tooth on your upper right side. You can use this position to floss as far as the cuspid on the upper left side. It is easier to move your lips out of the way if you open your jaw only as wide as you need in order to get your finger inside your mouth.

UPPER LEFT SIDE

1. To floss the left side, you do everything the same as when you floss the right side, except in reverse. Switch your hands so that your left hand is now held in front of your right hand, the floss is over the pad of your left thumb (braced with the index finger) and your right index finger, and the right index finger is now in your mouth. This changes the position of the floss.

2. Use this position to reach the last six teeth on the upper left side. Try this position between the central and lateral teeth on the upper left side before you work on the back ones. Let out more floss between your finger and thumb if you need more to reach the last teeth.

Flossing the lower jaw   I know, it's a trip learning how to floss the upper teeth, and I'm proud of you for hanging in there. Now I can give you some good news: learning how to floss the lower teeth is much easier. And soon you won't have to read about flossing anymore.

1. Wrap the floss around your right middle finger as you did when you flossed the upper teeth. Place the floss over the soft part of your right index finger. Pinch the loose end between your left thumb and index finger and pull it tight by separating your hands. Leave one inch to one and a half inches of floss between your hands.

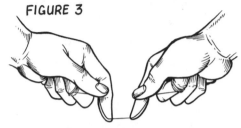

FIGURE 3

2. Then, starting from the lower left side, insert the finger-held floss into your mouth, and floss from the lower left to the lower right side. Are you getting the hang of it? See figure 3.

Flossing the backs of your teeth In a normal mouth there are four teeth with exposed backs: two on the upper jaw and two on the lower. Most people were never told to floss these areas, but these areas need flossing as much as the areas between the teeth.

It's really pretty easy to do. Hold the floss between the thumb and index finger of both hands. Allow about one to two inches of floss between your hands. Adjust your fingers so that you can loop the floss around the back tooth. Each of the four teeth will require a different finger positioning, but because there are many ways to do this, I leave it up to you to find the position that works best. If you have lost any teeth you'll need to floss the two sides adjacent to the void.

Part 2: Flossing Movements

All your teeth should be flossed in the same way, so I describe flossing movements between only two teeth. Practice these movements between the bottom front teeth; that way you can see in the bathroom mirror if you are doing it correctly.

1. Guide the floss to the space between two front teeth.

2. Pull it to one side (against one of the teeth) and slide it down the side of that tooth. At the same time as you pull the floss down, use a back-and-forth shimmy movement.

This movement helps flatten the floss and allows you to slide by a tight contact more easily than if you tried to force it straight

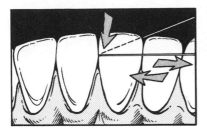

down through the contact point. This downward, shimmy movement also allows you to use less force. Not all contact points are the same. If you try to force the floss through a tight contact with a lot of pressure you can break the floss or snap it through the contact point, hitting the gums with a great deal of force. This can break the skin of the gums and cause bleeding, especially if you have infected gums.

3. Once you've passed the contact point, you're in what I call the "triangle area" between the teeth. The contact point is one point of the triangle, each tooth is one side of the triangle, and the gum between the teeth constitutes the third side. Every side of the triangle needs to be flossed.

Cleaning the teeth

1. Pull the floss against the side of one tooth and slide it up the tooth until it hits the contact point.

2. Wrap the floss around the tooth as far as you can. The size of your mouth and fingers determines how far you can wrap it.

3. Slide the floss down the tooth toward the gums, and make sure it goes as far down the tooth as it can go. This movement on the tooth is like shining the top of a shoe, with the floss as the polishing rag. Be careful not to jam the floss into the gums because it can injure them and force plaque into the pocket. Move the floss up and down six to eight times and then do the same to the opposite tooth.

4. Finish off each side with a few in-and-out movements. This in-and-out motion is very important, especially when you arrive at the junction of the tooth and gums, because it carries the food particles and plaque out into the mouth.

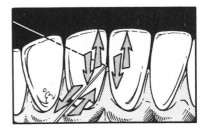

Cleaning the gums
After you have cleaned both sides of the triangle you need to massage the gums between your teeth. Be care-

ful if you have gum disease—the gums here may be very soft and fragile. Simply move the floss back and forth across the surface of the gums three or four times, exerting only slight pressure. This pressure massages the gums, helps toughen them, and increases blood flow. Increase the pressure as your gums become healthier, but never to the extent that they become sore and bleed.

Removing the floss How you remove the floss is critical. Since the day floss was invented, probably tens of thousands of fillings have been pulled out by improper floss removal. (Heck, sometimes dentists use floss to remove a stubborn, temporarily placed crown.) If a filling has not been done properly and protrudes beyond the tooth's surface, floss that is pulled out through the contact point can catch on the overhang and rip, fray, or get stuck. If enough force is used it can pull the filling out. This is not fun and will require a visit to the dentist. The trick is to *never* remove the floss by pulling it through the contact point if either tooth has a filling that overhangs the tooth. It's better to let go of the end of the floss inside your mouth and pull it straight through the triangle, slowly, toward the outside. When you are proficient at flossing, you will be able to tightly hold the floss between the thumb and index finger inside your mouth, instead of wrapping it around your middle finger. This makes it easier to pull the floss out through problem areas.

Flossing Tips

□ Check for bleeding. Once a week check the floss after you pull it out. If there is bleeding, it will appear on the floss as a reddish-pink color. Some flosses are colored red—don't use them when you check for bleeding. If you see any sign of blood note its location, because not only do you need to let your hygienist know but you need to give that area more attention when you brush, floss, and irrigate. Wipe or rinse off the floss, or use a new piece, before going on to the next flossing area.

□ You can use floss to check out whether the margin of a filling fits as well as it should. If the floss hangs up or frays make a note and point it out to the hygienist and dentist. Ask if the margin can be smoothed. (If the floss gets frayed, use a new piece.)

☐ Floss after you have brushed and spit out the excess paste, but before you have rinsed. The paste remaining between the teeth acts as a cleansing and polishing agent.

WATER IRRIGATION

You already know how much I like the water irrigator, so it's time to tell you who should use it, when, and how.

Who Should Use It

Anyone who has gum disease, especially if there's been bone loss, should always supplement their brushing and flossing with the use of a water irrigation device. But it's also a great preventive device and should be used even if you don't have gum disease.

When to Use It

If you have gum disease you should use it after you've brushed and flossed. After the disease has healed, use it at night, after your last brushing and flossing. But since it feels so refreshing, you may want to irrigate any old time.

How to Use It

Make a practice run without water in the container. Do this so that you can see your technique in the mirror and also to get the sensation of how the tip of the oral irrigator feels next to the gums. You can't do this if water is squirting all over the place. First read through the directions, and then run through the motions.

Begin at your regular starting place and follow the same pattern as you do when you brush. By now you should have this down pat. Make two or three complete passes through your mouth to perfect the technique.

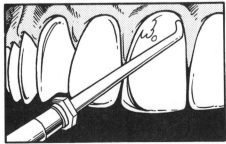

Adjust the tip of the irrigator so that it touches the area where the gum meets the tooth. Direct the tip so it is at an angle of forty-five degrees to the tooth. Make sure it is in direct contact with the gum line so that the jet of water has access to the gum pocket. If you have bone loss and spaces between your teeth, be sure and move the tip between the teeth and direct the water into the pocket on the sides of the teeth. Make the necessary adjustments as you move around the teeth. As you practice this, watch your movements in the mirror and tune in to how it feels, because when the water is shooting out your lips will be closed and you won't be able to see how you are doing. Irrigating is definitely a technique that relies on touch and feel.

The manufacturer of your water irrigation device will include directions on the use of its product. Each will have unique features, so be sure to read the directions.

How much time to spend The severity of the disease and the pocket depths on your periodontal chart will guide you as to the amount of time you need to spend. You should spend extra time in any area that has a pocket depth of 3 mm or more. The deeper the pocket, the more time you will spend.

Slowly move from tooth to tooth, and when you get to a problem area, stay there and move the tip back and forth along the gum line for five to ten seconds, then move on. If an area is not healing, spend more time at each session until it responds. As you increase the pressure, the liquid will run out faster, and in order to finish the job, you may have to refill the container.

Setting the water pressure The healthier your gums, the higher you can adjust the pressure setting. But if you have gum disease always start out on the lowest setting. Every three or four days you can move it up one notch, unless you have some spots that will require a lower setting for a longer period of time. The only way you can harm your gums using a water irrigation system is if you use too much water pressure before the gums have healed. Err on the side of too little pressure to begin with and be patient.

The liquid The liquid you use in the irrigator should always be close to body temperature. This is a must if you have had bone loss and/or sensitive teeth. To test the water, stick your finger in it, and if it feels neither cool nor warm it is at body temperature (when a liquid is 98.6°F you actually feel nothing). If you have gum disease use an antibacterial mouthwash or a saltwater solution with your irrigation device. *Note:* Be sure to check the product instructions to see if the manufacturer warns you against using any solution other than water.

Here are four ways to include mouthwash or a saline solution in your irrigator program (following the directions above with each method):

1. Fill the container with half mouthwash and half water.

2. Fill the container with water, and when you have used all the water, add two to three inches of undiluted mouthwash to finish off.

3. Use straight mouthwash. I recommend straight mouthwash if you are treating advanced periodontal disease. Also use straight mouthwash immediately after you have had hygiene therapy. This procedure keeps the germs in control until the gums have had a chance to recover.

4. If, for whatever reason, you're unable to use a mouthwash and don't have a problem with sodium, use a saltwater mixture. Salt is also very good for healing infection and has some antibacterial action. Use about one-half teaspoon of salt to a full container of body-temperature water. Stir it well. When your hygienist has declared you disease-free, and you're practicing preventive maintenance, back off on the salt or mouthwash solutions if you so desire.

Using straight mouthwash or a 50-percent mouthwash solution, although more expensive, is more effective than saltwater or plain water. The saltwater mix will produce good results, but sodium may not be advisable for some people. Using only water is about half as effective as the above methods, but will still reduce plaque and gingivitis more effectively than rinsing with plain water.

Keeping the liquid in check First, point the irrigator tip at the sink, turn on the irrigator, then let it run for a few seconds. This gets rid of the cold water left in the system after the last use. Shut it off, place the tip in your mouth next to the first tooth in your pattern, gently close your lips over the tip, then turn on the motor. If you forget to close your mouth water will spray all over the place. Lean over the sink, and when the water builds up in your mouth, simply tilt closer to the sink, open your lips a smidgen, and let the water run out. When the water has been released, close your mouth again and continue where you left off. When you do it this way you won't have to shut the irrigator off each time you release the water. You'll quickly get the hang of this.

Cleaning the Machine

If you use only water you won't have to clean the irrigator. If you mix anything else with the water, especially salt, you will *always* have to flush it out after you finish so the system won't become clogged. First, rinse out the container with fairly hot water. Then add a few inches of water to the container, turn to the highest setting (the water will run through faster), and run all the water through the tip. That's all there is to it.

Water Irrigator Tips

When deciding which irrigating system to purchase, you should take into consideration the size of the tip. If possible buy the one that offers the smallest tip. If the diameter of the tip is small enough you'll actually be able to gently insert it into the pocket. The further the liquid reaches into the pocket the better the results will be. This is especially valuable if you have pockets deeper than 4 mm. Always use gentle pressure, and never force the irrigator tip beyond a comfortable location. You could injure the gum tissue by forcing the tip into the pocket. It may be easier to gain access to a diseased pocket because the gum does not hold so tightly to the tooth. The new Pik Pocket Subgingival Tip by Teledyne Water Pik is the best small tip I've found.

TOOTHPICKS

Picks are probably the easiest to use of all the dental tools, especially the picks that have handles. But like everything on this planet, they, too, can be misused. The purpose of any pick is to break up plaque formation on the teeth, remove food particles, and massage and stimulate the gums in the gingival crevice area. Think of the pick as a miniature toothbrush that specializes in cleaning and massaging the vulnerable space between the tooth and the gum and the areas in between the teeth. For hard-to-reach areas, like the insides of all the teeth and the outsides of the back teeth, the size of the fingers makes regular toothpicks difficult to use. Picks that have small handles are much easier to control and will give better results.

How to Use Them

Hold the pick at a forty-five-degree angle to the gum line and gently place it into the gingival crevices. Don't force it into the pocket; you might injure the tissue. Practice positioning the pick on the front teeth and check yourself in the mirror. All you have to do is angle the pick as shown in the drawing.

Move around the crev- ice using the same pattern you use when you brush, be- ginning with the last tooth on the side you've chosen. When you've cleaned every area, rinse your mouth well with water. If you're at home 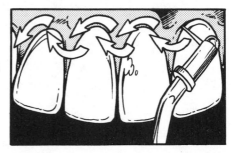 it will be more effective to use an oral irrigator because it will really wash away all the plaque and food stirred up by the picking.

Pick Tips

- ☐ If you use a wooden toothpick, nibble on the point until you have blunted it and created a frayed, brushlike end. This will keep you from accidentally penetrating the skin, and the frayed end acts like a miniature brush. If you use a plastic pick watch out. Some of them have sharp points. Lightly sand the tip with fine sandpaper until the point is no longer sharp.

- ☐ If you have periodontal disease you can soak the end of your frayed toothpick in mouthwash or hydrogen peroxide (a 3 percent solution). Stim-U-Dents also work well with these antibacterial agents. You will not only mechanically dislodge the plaque but also add chemical germ fighters.

- ☐ Get one of the handy toothpick holders and always keep it with you. Or else use regular toothpicks. But whatever your choice, if you can't brush or floss after eating, at least pick.

DISCLOSING AGENTS

Disclosing agents come with directions for their use, but I would like to add my own two-cents-worth. If you use them while you're in the process of learning your new hygiene techniques, it will be almost like having your hygienist come home with you to point out where you're cleaning well and where you're not. If you use tablets let them dissolve in your mouth before you brush. If you use the liquid just swish it thoroughly around your teeth. Use your mouth mirror to check for the stains that indicate food and plaque. Then go through your brushing pattern and take another look. Then floss and take another peek. Then use the water irrigator and take a final gander. You will see that each successive procedure has removed more of the stained food and plaque.

Using disclosing agents is one of the best ways to demonstrate the effects of proper oral hygiene techniques, especially to children. During the early stages of its formation, plaque is impossible to see with the unaided eye. This makes it difficult to conceptualize. That old but-if-I-can't-see-it-how-can-it-be-there attitude is not the right attitude to take. But once plaque is stained with a disclosing agent (and it stains very well), you have visual proof that it exists. Keep using disclosing agents periodically, say once a week, while establishing your hygiene program, until you see that you are no longer missing any areas. After that you can use it every few months as a monitor.

RINSING AND GARGLING

Rinsing and gargling are not the same. They are not performed the same way, and they do not produce the same results. Try a little experiment. I call it the rinse-versus-gargle experiment. Do it after you eat your most complete meal of the day. If you add beets to your meal the results will be even more spectacular. First, brush, floss, and irrigate your mouth as you normally would. Then, rinse with water, but don't gargle. You would think that after these procedures all food particles would be washed away. Well, I suggest that there is an area you've missed, and here's how to find out where that is.

Make sure the sink is clean, then stop it up. Next, take a small swig of water. Tilt your head back and gargle real well: deep, high, and long. (You might need to experiment with the amount of water needed to both gargle and avoid a gag reflex.) The head tilting is critical, as it allows the water to move farther back into the throat, which is what distinguishes gargling from rinsing. Experiment and work the water as far back in your throat as you can before doing the actual gargling. With practice you will reach areas in the back of your throat you never thought you could. Spit the gargled water into the sink and take a look at what you've found. What do you see? I thought so!

The back part of the mouth and the upper part of the throat act as a catchall for many of the foods we eat. The foods that are especially troublesome are mucous-forming foods, such as dairy products, flour products, foods to which you may be allergic, and foods that contain sugar. It is possible that some of the food that sticks to the palate and upper throat will find its way back to the teeth and gums, perhaps when you clear your throat or cough. Why put in all that time on oral hygiene and then have food particles sneak in through the back door?

There are other reasons to gargle after brushing. One is that when food particles, particularly dairy products and foods containing sugar, start hanging out in the back of your throat, they provide a super breeding ground for all kinds of bacteria. Left there long enough, these toxic little germs will breed faster than the proverbial rabbit. In large numbers they can create enough irritation and infection to cause sore throats, and I believe they are a contributing cause of strep throat. I also think that this environment plays a role in the development of tonsillitis. The lymph system that protects the upper throat and back of the mouth can be overwhelmed and weakened from constantly fighting off these germs and the irritation and toxins they produce.

Another reason to gargle is to get rid of excess bacteria and food particles that could cause unwelcome bad breath. So do your immune system, your throat, your teeth and gums, and your friends' noses a favor: add both rinsing and gargling to your daily oral hygiene program.

Even if you can't brush or floss after eating, you should both rinse and gargle. When you rinse be sure to suck the water back and forth between the teeth, particularly if you have had bone loss. Wherever you have had bone loss and gum recession there will be gaps between the teeth where the gums once lived. Passive rinsing will not reach these areas as well as forceful sucking will. Boy, that old bone loss really comes back to haunt you.

CLEANING THE TONGUE

If you're like most people, you may not have been giving your tongue much attention, but the tongue needs to be cleaned as much as the teeth do. From the germ's point of view the tongue is the perfect place to live. The taste buds are like trees that snag food and protect germs from brushing, flossing, and rinsing. You could be doing a super cleaning job on your teeth and still have a high oral germ count because the tongue is not being cleaned.

There are two ways of cleaning the tongue. The first is to clean it with the toothbrush. Rinse your brush with warm water, stick your tongue out as far as you can, put your brush as far back on the tongue as you can without going into the gag reflex, and brush it from back to front. I have found that using a 2-by-2-inch gauze strip to grasp the slippery tip of your tongue keeps it from slipping away. Brush with as much pressure as you can tolerate, but don't abuse it. There are thousands of sensitive taste buds residing there. Rinse the brush after each pass over the tongue.

The second way is to clean it with a teaspoon. I find it easier to use than the brush. First, rinse a clean spoon under warm water. When it has reached body temperature, open your mouth, stick out your tongue, and place the spoon, with the concave side down, as far back on the tongue as you can without gagging. Press the spoon against the tongue and drag it lightly toward the tip of the tongue. Check the contents of the spoon. How about that? Your tongue is one of the body's measuring sticks: the better your diet and the healthier you are, the cleaner the spoon will be.

You might try using both techniques: brush it first, and then finish cleaning your tongue with the spoon. Remember to be gentle, but clean as much of it as you can.

SPECIAL SITUATIONS

There are very few ideal mouths—mouths that contain perfectly straight teeth with no decay or periodontal disease. So since most of us have some sort of oral idiosyncrasy, I'll pass along a few tips for dealing with special problems that are often overlooked.

Misaligned Teeth

If you have overlapping teeth the areas where the teeth overlap will be more stained and junk-filled than areas where the teeth are straight. To verify this, look at your teeth after you have eaten some bread, seeds, or nuts. Note where the chewed food sticks and where it does not. Also, check those misaligned areas against your periodontal pocket depth chart. I bet you find that the gums here are not as healthy as the gums around the straight teeth.

Most brushing techniques are designed for straight teeth, and in order to compensate for overlapping teeth you must change the angle of the brush. You can't brush with the same up-and-down motion that you use in other areas. This is very important. If you don't compensate for the misalignment, you won't be able to effectively remove the food and plaque. Be creative with your brush and spend extra time in those areas. Flossing, water irrigating, and picking are also a *must* in these areas.

Missing Teeth

Missing teeth create unique brushing problems. You'll have to pay special attention not only to the teeth on either side of the space left by the lost tooth but also to the tooth above or below the space. Because the tooth directly above or below no longer has a partner, it is more vulnerable to decay and gum disease; the natural self-cleansing process that is a by-product of chewing no longer exists for that tooth. Until you get the missing tooth replaced, I recommend that you use either a small children's brush or one with a specialized head to clean around the teeth next to the empty space. And don't forget to floss and irrigate these areas.

Margins

Margin is the dental term for the place where a filling meets the tooth. It may be easier for you to think of margins as joints or seams. Whatever you decide to call them, these areas are highly vulnerable to plaque formation and thus to decay, especially the margins of a filling found between the teeth. From a germ's perspective, a margin is as wide as the Grand Canyon. If germs can penetrate a healthy tooth, you know they sure as heck can weasel their way into the space between a filling and the tooth. And they can do it even more easily if the filling does not fit tightly or if it overhangs the place where it meets the tooth. Make sure you give special hygiene attention to every tooth that has a filling, especially crowns and composite restorations. The amalgam filling is more resistant to re-decay because germs don't like mercury but they still need attention.

Fixed Bridges

Everyone knows that artificial teeth do not decay, so you might be wondering why they have to be kept clean. Well, plaque and calculus can form on all man-made materials placed in your mouth. Even well-constructed crowns and fixed bridges create food and plaque traps, and they aren't as easily cleaned by the chewing process as are your natural teeth. If they are not properly cared for, plaque can form rapidly, and calculus formation won't be far behind. It won't take long for the plaque to reach the gums around the false tooth (called a *pontic*), irritating them and causing inflammation. The plaque that forms on the bridge itself also acts as a breeding ground and food storage area for germs and can be a contributing cause of decay, gum disease, and bad breath. The brush will not reach all the areas of the bridge that need cleaning, so you must use a floss threader to get the floss between the pontic and the gum to clean every area you 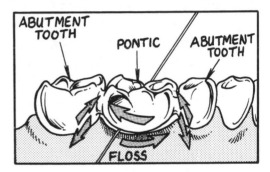 can reach. Make sure you floss the sides of the natural teeth next to the pontic. The shaded areas in the drawing indicate where you need to floss, at least once a day. Use the water irrigator to rinse away the stuff you've loosened and to massage the gum underneath the pontic.

Removable Dental Appliances

These are commonly referred to as *partial dentures*. If you don't take care of them they can become just as dirty as uncared-for natural teeth. Special attention should be paid to the areas where the partial attaches to the natural teeth. The natural teeth that hold and support the partial, called *abutments*, undergo a great deal of stress. They are also major food and plaque traps. Because they are so important you should consciously zero in on them and give them as much care and time as it takes to keep them healthy. Always ask your RDH to give you a report on how well you are doing in those vulnerable areas. Without proper care you could lose an abutment tooth, and the partial could have to be remade. You may already know how expensive that is.

Full or Half Dentures

Dentures and denture care are covered in Chapter 15.

Braces (Orthodontic Appliances)

Braces have come a long way since their introduction, but keeping them clean is just as important today as it was thirty years ago. For as much good as they do, they're also germ and plaque traps. Therefore you must spend extra time brushing around the areas where the braces are attached.

Always brush and irrigate both the top and bottom portions of the braces. Think of the braces as the gingival crevice and use the same circular shimmy motion and you'll do fine. Because you can't floss with braces, you'll have to make up for that loss with extra brushing and, especially, use of the water irrigator. Kids find this a fun thing to do . . . and when any task is fun it's performed more often. When using the irrigator,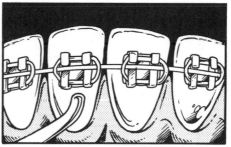

IRRIGATOR TIP

make sure that you direct the jet of water from the top down and from the bottom up. The electric toothbrush is great for cleaning braces. Avoiding foods that germs love—substituting lots of raw vegetables and fruit in place of soft, processed, and refined foods, especially junk food—is especially important when braces are involved.

TIPS FOR THE DISABLED

If you have problems with or have lost the use of your hands, oral hygiene is not so easy. Hopefully, you have a friend or a loved one who can assist you with your dental care. If you have artificial limbs the electric toothbrush (especially the Panasonic Powerfloss brush with its power flosser), water irrigator, and floss holder will be invaluable. I strongly recommend that you pay strict attention to your diet: diet is the most natural of all the tools available. Read the chapter on nutrition (Chapter 16) for detailed information. Avoid sugar, use a mouthwash, and top off your meals with carrots and apples. Have your teeth cleaned often—your dental hygienist will help you determine a cleaning schedule. Our newsletter will keep you updated about the latest tools and techniques for the disabled.

DR. TOM'S TIPS

I wasn't always a dentist. I was a patient first, and not a very good one, at that. By the time I was eighteen, I had chronic gingivitis around many teeth and the beginnings of periodontitis around a few others. My parents took me to the dentist every six months, and though it helped, I was still on my way to becoming a dental cripple. For me, getting back on track was a process of turning my bad dental habits (more like no dental habits) into teeth-saving ones. But I found that even after I learned all the hows and whys of dental prevention and oral hygiene, some of my old habits remained.

For those of you finding it difficult to change old and unproductive habits, I'd like to pass along a few of the things that helped me change. Over the years I developed several novel ways to make my oral hygiene more effective. So if you want to establish new hygiene habits I suggest you at least give them a try.

☐ When you're sure that you've mastered the basic techniques of oral hygiene, try adding some variety to your program. You would be surprised at how much exercise you can do while brushing your teeth and gums. I like to do stretching and toning exercises. The stretches I find easy and fun to do are side bends, leg raises, toe lifts, twists, squats, and other forms of isotonic exercise. Feel free to create your own exercises. This is a great way to get rid of decay and burn some calories at the same time. You can also think of it the other way around: while you're exercising throw in a little hygiene.

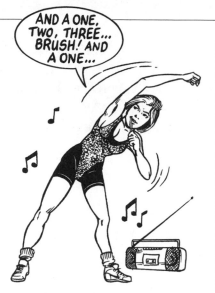

☐ Brush and floss in the shower. Why not clean your mouth and body at the same time? I don't use toothpaste when I brush in the shower, but there's no reason you can't. Rinsing after you brush is a breeze (no toothpaste on the shirt or blouse), and the shower head acts as an oral irrigator and helps to clean and massage the gums.

☐ If you like to read try it while cleaning your teeth and gums. Over a period of a year, those few minutes a day really add up. I keep a book about music theory in my bathroom. A friend of mine uses that time every day to learn Spanish. But I should warn you now that trying to read while flossing does not work too well, unless you have a bookstand.

If you're worrying about whether you can brush too much, don't. I have yet to see a problem that has resulted from brushing or flossing too much, once patients have learned the right technique. But I have seen thousands of patients who have developed serious dental problems from not brushing enough. You can choose the side of the coin you prefer. When it comes to saving your teeth, any approach is worth a try. What have you got to lose? . . . except your teeth.

You may come up with other suggestions for making it more fun and less of a chore to take care of your mouth. If you do I'd appreciate hearing from you. Write to me at the address in the Appendix, and I'll pass your ideas along to your fellow dental patients via *The Tooth Fitness Digest*.

HYGIENE AWAY FROM HOME

Most people have what I call "neutral time" during the day. These are times when you are alone—thinking, walking, sitting, watching TV, driving. Taking advantage of these times to work on your oral hygiene not only saves time in the bathroom but makes it easier to keep your mouth in perfect health. I don't know about you, but the less time I have to spend in the bathroom taking care of my teeth, the happier I am. If you feel the same way, you may find these tips helpful.

Floss and Picks

Always carry floss and picks or have them handy. Floss and picks are the easiest of all the tools to carry and use. I have a container of floss in my car, in the drawer in my office, and in my little day pack. After I developed the right habits, I found that a little floss alarm would go off in my brain at certain times of the day, after I ate, when I'd go for my walk, and while I was lying in bed. Besides flossing in the morning and at night before bed, make sure that you floss at least one other time—after lunch is ideal. Don't just think in terms of numbers, like twice a day—think in terms of opportunity. Floss whenever you can, and if it turns out to be four or five times a day, so much the better. When it's done correctly, you can never floss too much!

Automobile Hygiene

If you commute to work, either as a driver or a passenger, you can cut down on bathroom time by making the car a mobile hygiene center. Keep both floss and a pick holder in your car at all times. Get into the habit of flossing and using the pick every time you have to wait for a traffic light and whenever you're stuck in traffic. You may not finish a full cycle at each stop signal, so just remember where you left off and start from there at the next light. Don't snicker—some poor folks get stuck in commuter traffic as much as two hours a day, and this time can add up to hundreds of hours of positive hygiene. Listening to music may be good for the spirits, but it won't save a single tooth. So put on your favorite tape—and floss and pick away at every opportunity.

Finger Brushing

When nothing else is available you can use your index finger as a brush. Although your finger doesn't have bristles, massaging your gums this way is better than nothing.

SOMETHING TO THINK ABOUT

Taking care of your mouth should not be a struggle. After experimenting with my suggestions you'll find that the time you spend brushing seems to fly by, and you'll actually enjoy doing something that is good for you. Don't look at taking care of your mouth as something you *have* to do but rather as something that you *get* to do. After all, there are over 13 million Americans who wish they had some teeth to take care of. I hope you will never know how miserable it is not to have your own teeth. Every time you brush, floss, irrigate, pick, and have your teeth cleaned, you increase the odds of keeping them. With the proper care, your teeth can accompany you on your journey from the cradle to the grave. Keeping them will be up to you,

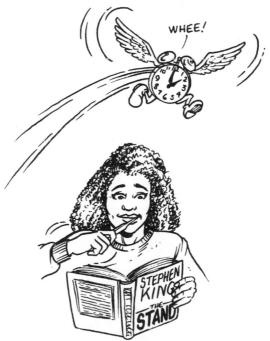

WHEE!

not just your dentist or your hygienist, so you might as well enjoy the oral hygiene process. Look at it this way: *You certainly do not have to take care of all of your teeth all of the time—only the ones you want to keep.*

YOUR HOME CARE CHECKLIST

☐ Establish your hygiene pattern.

☐ Brush after every meal if possible, but for sure in the morning and the evening.

☐ Floss after every brushing if possible, and whenever else you can, but always before you go to bed.

☐ Rinse and gargle after brushing and flossing, and after every meal, especially if you can't brush and floss.

☐ Chew sugarless gum if you can't brush after eating foods containing sugar.

☐ Irrigate after your last brushing and flossing of the day.

☐ Use picks anytime, but especially after eating if you can't brush.

☐ Clean your tongue daily or as often as you can.

PART TWO

The Dental Team and You

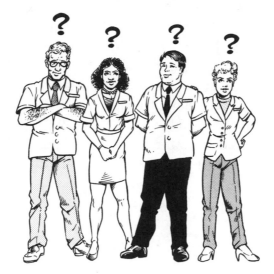

Chapter 6

Finding a Dentist and a Dental Hygienist

If you don't have a regular dentist, or if you are looking for a new one, this chapter will help you find one. If you already have a dentist and a dental hygienist with whom you feel comfortable you can skip this and go on to the next chapter.

FINDING A DENTIST

Finding just any dentist is about as easy as breathing or falling off a log. Finding the right one for you is not so easy, but with a little effort, it can be done. Dentists are not stamped out like robots; though some people may disagree, they are actually human beings. As such, they have different personalities and different attitudes and approaches to repair, prevention, and their patients. And they are not all the same when it comes to the quality of their repair work—some are definitely better than others. But it's not enough just to find one who does high-quality repair work. The ultimate success of your oral hygiene program will hinge on your finding a dentist who not only is conscientious about his work but also sincerely cares about your oral health—a dentist you trust and with whom you can get along and *who supports your total preventive program.*

If you follow my guidelines it should not be difficult to find a dentist who cares about you, treats you well, does high-quality dental repair, and is fully committed to prevention. The key to any lasting dental treatment is, and will always be, prevention. So if you find yourself with a dentist who can't seem to find the time for prevention, or who thinks it has gone the way of the dinosaur, immediately start the search for another one who knows and appreciates its importance. Don't settle for less. There are plenty of dentists who are happy to treat the whole patient, not just the teeth that need repair.

Keep in mind that surgery is being performed on your body when you have your teeth drilled and filled or extracted, when you have implants (see Chapter 15), and when you undergo certain periodontal procedures. Dentistry is actually a special branch of medicine, and the same rights and responsibilities that apply to the medical patient apply to the dental patient. You have the right to get a second opinion if it is needed, and even to change dentists if you are not satisfied. You also have the right (and indeed, the responsibility) to do whatever it takes to find a dentist you can trust.

Most people don't think twice about seeking out two or three bids when it comes to hiring an electrician or a building contractor. Yet far too many people, erroneously believing all dentists are alike, browse through the phone book and randomly choose a dentist. There are better ways, without relying on the element of chance, to find a dentist who will be right for you.

Word of Mouth

Asking friends and acquaintances for a recommendation is a very effective way to find a dentist. With friends, not only are you able to ask intimate questions about their personal dental experiences but you are also likely to receive truthful answers. In this way, you'll have a better chance of hearing about dentists whom you should avoid. It's important to ask a friend not only what he likes but also what he does not like about his dentist—it could be something you, too, may not like.

You don't have to limit your inquiries to friends, family, or business acquaintances. Even a perfect stranger, one who has a radiant, healthy smile, can lead you to your new dentist. If you want to ask a stranger about his or her dentist and nothing comes to mind, try this: "Hi, you sure have a beautiful smile. Mind if I ask the name of your dentist?" This could also be a good opening line to use if you want to meet someone. Who knows, you could meet your future spouse and find a dentist at the same time! Regardless of whom you contact, you should ask all of the following questions:

☐ Does your dentist have an active prevention program?

☐ Do you *trust* him and have confidence in his abilities?

☐ Is he concerned about you, and do you feel supported by him?

☐ Can you ask him questions easily?

☐ Does he explain things clearly and in a way that you can understand?

☐ Is the office staff pleasant and courteous?

☐ Have you had any problem with the work your dentist has done for you?

☐ Do you honestly like him, or would you rather be going to someone else?

Communicate with the Dental Profession

Contact dental hygienists   The dental hygienist might be the best source of information when you're searching for a dentist with a holistic approach to dentistry. That is, if you can get one to give you information. Hygienists have to watch their p's and q's when recommending dentists. The dentist for whom the hygienist works will not be a happy camper if he finds out that she's sent a patient to another dentist. But it's worth the effort to get her advice because she probably knows more about the dentist's repair skills, personality, work ethic, and attitude toward prevention than anyone else, including the dentist's family. In addition, most hygienists work for more than one dentist, and they have hygienist friends who work for other dentists. They can be a gold mine of information.

If you know a hygienist the best place to ask her your questions is anywhere away from the office. If you must ask her while you're at the dental office, be very subtle. When you're alone with her, casually ask who does her own dental work. Asking in this way gets her off the hook because you're not specifically asking her to recommend someone. You may come up with a better way to ask her, but whatever your approach, don't pass up this great opportunity. However, if she is unwilling, don't press her. Instead, ask her the phone number of the local dental hygiene association, and ask them to refer you to a quality dentist who has a prevention-oriented practice.

Contact dental specialists   All dental specialists rely heavily on the general dentist for patient referral. They see a lot of patients and have a good idea about the ability of each dentist. Not every specialist will be willing to give you a recommendation though. Some may be concerned that by referring a patient to one dentist, they will create bad "public relations" with the others. But it isn't unethical for them to offer referrals, and it's worth a try to obtain one.

If the direct approach doesn't work you can try another approach. Dental specialists have mouths, too, and that means they also have dentists. And believe me, when they pick one, they pick a good one. An auto mechanic can work on his own car, but I've never heard of a dentist who works on his own teeth. So if you're seeing a dental specialist for any reason and don't have a regular dentist, or want to find a new one, this is the question to ask: "Who do you see for your own dental work?" If you're not seeing a specialist you can call the office of any specialist listed in the telephone book and ask his receptionist for the name of a general dentist their office recommends. Don't bother her with specific questions, just get the name. She may not know anything else about him, anyway, except that he has a good reputation at their office.

Contact your current dentist   This applies if you're moving, or are planning to move, to another town and are satisfied with your current dentist. Dentists know other dentists. Over the years your dentist will have met many dentists from other parts of the state and country. Although there's no guarantee that Dr. George in San Francisco will personally know of a dentist in Big Timber, Montana, there's a surprisingly good chance that he will. If you've already moved and still haven't found a dentist that fills the bill, give your old dentist a call.

Inquire at Dental Schools

If you live in a large city there may be a dental school in your area. Check the yellow pages for the number of the local dental association, listed under Dental Referral Services. Call and ask if there is a dental school in your area. If there is, you can call the school and ask them to refer you to a general dentist with a private practice who also teaches at the school. Though there are always exceptions, many of the dentists who take the time and financial loss in order to

DR. TOM'S TIPS

Most people are not aware of this, but dental schools provide dental treatment. Dental students, under direct supervision, work on patients. There are three advantages to this.

☐ The first is low cost. Whatever work is done in the dental school will be significantly less expensive than having the same work done in the dental office.

☐ The second advantage is the good quality of the work. The students are overseen and graded on every step of each procedure, so the caliber of the work is very good. How well they perform in the dental school clinic will help determine whether or not they graduate. The only instructors that dentists in private practice have standing over their shoulders are their consciences. For most dentists, having a good conscience is enough of a monitor, but not for all.

☐ The third advantage is that most dental schools have graduate programs in which dentists are taught to do advanced work. In those programs, quality advanced work in areas such as periodontics, orthodontics, implants, and oral and maxillofacial surgery is available at a reasonable cost.

Alas, there is a flip side to this shiny coin. The big disadvantage of being a dental school patient is that your dental work will take more time. And, technically, you haven't found a dentist, more like a soon-to-be dentist, but if you have the time and patience, want good work, and want to save money, it's a pretty good deal.

teach are people who care. They also are probably up-to-date on the latest techniques, equipment, and materials and are likely to add them to their own practices. But there are no guarantees that you will get the perfect dentist, so you will still have to see if he meets your individual requirements. The dental school is also a good place to find a dental specialist, from the oral surgeon to the orthodontist.

Use the Yellow Pages

Twenty years ago, if you looked for a dentist in the telephone book you would find only his name, phone number, address, and individual speciality. Fortunately, dentists are now advertising their services, and that makes it easy for you to see if they fill your requirements. While it is true that you should take everything you hear or read with a grain of salt, the yellow pages are still a good place from which to start.

The information the telephone book supplies can save you from dialing number after number only to ask each receptionist to identify the aspects of dentistry the dentist emphasizes. To see what I mean, take a minute and look at the advertisements in the yellow pages listed under Dentists. How many general dentists mention prevention? You'll discover that a majority of them do not. I don't know about you, but it definitely makes me wonder. If a dentist advertises, it means to me that he wants you to know what he emphasizes, what he does well, and what he thinks is important. And if he doesn't tell the world that he stresses prevention, just how impor-

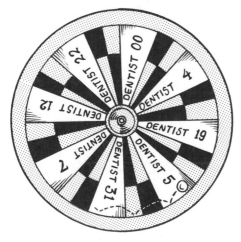

tant can he really think it is? That he omits prevention from his advertising doesn't necessarily mean that he doesn't care about it or stress it or that he's not a good dentist. However, if you are using only the yellow pages to select your dentist, why take a chance—choose one who includes prevention in his advertisement.

Dial 800-DENTIST

This free 800 number is another way to find yourself a dentist. You should know that the dentist being recommended is a member of the American Dental Association, is paying for the privilege of being listed with this service, and probably has written his own resume. It is useful to find out what he thinks about himself, but I'd hardly consider it an impartial evaluation. And just because a dentist is a member of the ADA doesn't mean that he does better work than a nonmember, that he's a nice guy, or that he's a strong supporter of preventive education.

When you call this number you can ask specific questions; thus it is a step up from looking through the yellow pages. (The yellow pages can be valuable, but they cannot speak.) While such a service can help you in your search for a dentist, it only goes so far. A listing does not guarantee a dentist's work, and your choice of a particular dentist will still come down to how you feel about him.

FINDING A DENTAL HYGIENIST

In a sense, it is easier to find an RDH because you'll get her when you get your dentist. But if your present hygienist isn't the one for you or you're looking for one for the first time, here's how you go about finding one.

- ☐ Find a dentist whose office stresses prevention. This will usually mean that the hygienist has been allowed to design a good preventive program for the dentist's patients. This is critical, because if the dentist isn't into prevention the hygienist's hands may be tied: she may not be allowed to spend the necessary time to develop, and then follow up on, an effective oral hygiene program. *Simply scraping and polishing your teeth should never be considered all there is to preventive dentistry.* When you find the right dentist you will probably be blessed with the right hygienist.

- ☐ If for some reason you don't have a dentist, don't want one, and only want to see a hygienist, you can talk to your friends. Ask them the same questions you would ask if you were looking for a dentist. There is no law against seeing a hygienist without also seeing a dentist. But, while seeing only a hygienist may be better than not seeing either one, I *do not* recommend it. Even though I've said this ad nauseam, I must say it one more time: if you really want to eliminate dental disease you'll need both of them working for you. She may be the hygiene expert, but she doesn't diagnose disease or repair teeth.

ONCE YOU HAVE FOUND A DENTIST

Once you've done the investigative work and have the name of a dentist, you've taken an important first step. But there's more—confirming that you've made a good choice. Below are two checklists. The first lists questions to ask the office receptionist when you first call the office. The second provides some guidelines as to what to look for after you have found your way to the dental office. These checklists are not meant as a strict test for the dentist, but as an aid for you.

You can evaluate some of the items on the second checklist at your first visit; others will take more time. You must also take into account the intangibles that you can sense by feeling and intuition. You must make up your own mind, but remember that no one is perfect, and even if the dentist and his staff do not hit 100 percent, it doesn't mean they won't be perfect for you.

When You Call for the First Appointment

The following are some questions to ask the receptionist when you call the office. They will make your dental visits better, for both you and the dental staff.

☐ What should you should expect on your first visit? Should you bring anything with you? Your insurance forms, X rays from your previous office, etc.?

☐ Does the office handle the paperwork for insurance? Dental offices are not obligated to provide this service, and not all of them do. Dealing with dental insurance can be difficult and time-consuming if you don't know what you are doing. Dental offices understand insurance forms, and this service is a definite advantage because their help can save you time and money as well as making sure you receive all the benefits you're entitled to.

☐ Does the dentist have a policy of seeing emergency patients immediately? You may never have an emergency, but you need to know if your dentist will make himself available to you if you do.

There are also things you should tell the receptionist:

☐ Let her know if you think you have a tooth or gum problem that, while not an emergency, may need prompt treatment. That way you can be scheduled in such a way as to accommodate your needs and avoid disrupting the rest of the patients' appointments. They'll appreciate you for that kindness.

☐ Let her know if you have any ailments or disabilities that could affect the amount of time you can spend at the office.

What to Look for When You Get There

☐ Is the office prevention-oriented?

☐ Is the office staff pleasant?

☐ Do they treat you like a human being, complete with intelligence and feelings, and not just like a mouth?

☐ Do they insist on taking a complete health history during your first visit, and do they update it at every hygiene recall appointment?

☐ Is the dentist personable?

☐ Does the dentist do a thorough oral examination?

☐ Does he recommend a full-mouth set of X rays before he designs your treatment plan? (Emergency appointments are an exception.)

☐ Does he offer you a complete treatment plan, one that includes the best treatment available, along with less expensive alternatives?

☐ Does the dentist usually work with a dental assistant?

☐ Are the injections mostly painless?

☐ After the initial work is finished, are your follow-up visits problem-free (fillings never fall out and the dentist never has to fill the same tooth over again)?

- ☐ Does the dentist suggest follow-up exams and regular hygiene therapy recalls?
- ☐ Would the dentist rather try to save a tooth than pull it?
- ☐ Does he seem relaxed and therefore make you feel that he has the time to give you the attention you deserve?
- ☐ Is the hygienist fully supportive of your prevention program?
- ☐ Are you encouraged to ask questions?
- ☐ Are your questions always answered to your satisfaction?
- ☐ Does the office practice effective infection control practices? (See Chapter 19 for specifics.)
- ☐ Is the office neat, clean, and comfortable?
- ☐ Is the equipment modern and well cared for?
- ☐ Did your dentist have a happy look on his face when he saw *Tooth Fitness* in your hand?

One last thought. Once you have found a dentist, and you are satisfied that he's the one for you, you need to know how to get the most out of him and the rest of the dental staff. The next three chapters will tell you how to do just that.

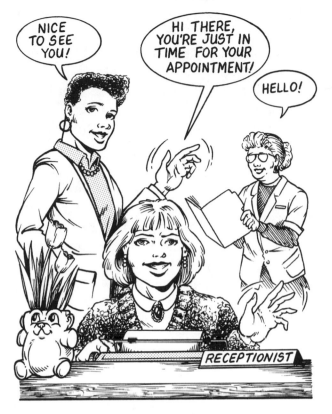

Chapter 7

The Front Office: Making It Work for You

Every visit to the dentist begins with the front office. But if you do not understand what the office staff does, you're not likely to appreciate how important they can be to your quest for oral health. They interact with a lot of people each day, and not all meetings are positive encounters. So make sure yours is one of the positive ones. Treat them with kindness and respect, and you can expect to get the same in return. Not only will they appreciate it, but they'll be on your side. They may go that extra mile to get you a better appointment time or be understanding when you are late on a payment. I've been backstage at the dental office, and I know what the staff talks about. I've heard things like, "Oh, no. That jerk Stan is coming in today. I'm definitely taking my break when he comes." Or, "Guess what? That nice Mrs. Sparks is scheduled this afternoon. I can't wait to see her. She's such a treat."

If you go out of your way to be nice to the front office team, and they don't respond in kind, it could be a reflection of the dentist's attitude . . . or it could just be their personalities. If you're happy with the dentist and everything else is working out, mention to the dentist how you are being treated, in a private meeting. It could be that the people in question are efficient and friendly to him but real ogres to the patients, and he may not be aware of it. It could be hurting his practice, and it would be important for him to know this. This approach makes sense only if you have been courteous and have done your part, such as showing up on time and paying your bills.

Depending on the size of the office, you could be dealing with one or all of the following: dental receptionist, office manager, and dental assistant.

THE RECEPTIONIST

The job of the receptionist is not an easy one, though it is made easier if the dentist for whom she works is a good and conscientious one. She has to be both thin- and tough-skinned to handle this job because, like an intersection, everyone goes through her first. She handles the scheduling of appointments, most of the phone calls, insurance and regular billing, and complaints, and gets too little praise in return. I suggest that when you talk to her in person at your first appointment, tell her what days and hours work best for you. You might not always get what you want, but you'll have a better chance. If you're in a hurry to have your work done and are having a difficult time getting scheduled, tell her that you would love to take the place of someone who has canceled. She'll put you on her cancellation list, and if you're flexible enough you will probably get in sooner and more often.

A good receptionist is a little like a therapist and is worth her weight in gold. Everyone likes to cry on her shoulder, including the dentist. You aren't the only patient she sees, but she has to treat you as if you are. Give her a "Well done" now and then.

THE OFFICE MANAGER

The office manager oversees the operation of the entire office and makes sure that it is running smoothly. She's the grease that keeps the gears turning. She's usually the most experienced of the front office staff and has cut her teeth, so to speak, as a receptionist. In a busy office she may help the receptionist and even do some dental assisting. Most receptionists and office managers have had dental assisting experience, so you can feel comfortable if she occasionally replaces the regular assistant. If your dentist has an office manager and you have any problems or questions about bills, scheduling, or personalities that the receptionist can't resolve, the front office manager is the one you should speak to.

THE ASSISTANT

Modern dentistry often requires four hands. Since every dentist I know has only two, the assistant has to supply the other two. The assistant also handles infection control, keeps track of supplies, takes X rays and impressions, places temporary fillings, and works with the receptionist on scheduling. In addition, assistants do about a hundred other things that help make your visit successful.

She provides valuable moral support and helps you deal with your fears and anxieties. But only if you let her know. She also acts as a kind of buffer between you and the dentist. She's great at passing on your concerns and questions. If there is anything you want to ask the dentist, but are hesitant or embarrassed, just pretend she is the dentist. In most cases she can answer the question, but if she can't she will get the answer for you. Remember, she isn't there only to help the dentist.

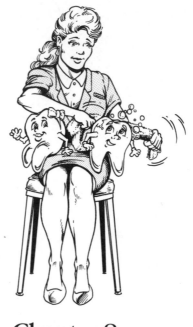

Chapter 8

Working with the Dental Hygienist

Because this book's main focus is prevention, this chapter is de-voted to the person who will, if you let her, play the most critical role in your overall preventive education program—the registered dental hygienist (RDH). (Many dentists perform hygiene therapy as well, so when I refer to the hygienist, I'm also including them.) You will discover what she does and why, as well as how to take full advantage of her knowledge and experience. Establishing a positive relationship with her could make the difference between a success-ful or unsuccessful hygiene program. And as with any harmonious relationship, both participants will benefit from it. So this chapter is also intended to help make your hygienist's work easier, and cer-tainly more rewarding. There are other sections in the book you may be able to browse through or skip entirely, but this is not one of them.

Your dental hygienist has undergone between two and four years of full-time, highly specialized training in order to provide you with this healing service. She is not a dentist, but she can certainly be called a preventive dental specialist. Not only is she qualified to perform hygiene therapy and to be a great source of preventive knowledge, but she is also your in-office oral guide and support person. When all is said and done, her primary role is to help you save your teeth. As the preventive expert of the dental team, her role is "to save them so the doc can fix them so you can smile and eat with them." It doesn't take a rocket scientist to figure out that no matter how good a dentist is at repair, he can't repair your teeth if you don't have them.

As your personal guide to preventive oral care, your RDH will be one of the best values you may ever get. You must have seen those commercials in which some dental aid is claimed to be the best there is for removing plaque and controlling calculus. Well, they all pale compared to her. No one fights plaque and calculus the way she does—not even your 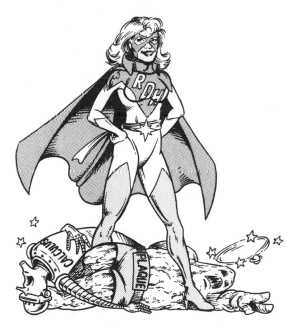 dentist. Batgirl can't hold a candle to Plaque Lady. You'd be awfully foolish not to take full advantage of what she offers.

WHAT YOUR HYGIENE THERAPIST DOES FOR YOU

Hygiene therapy used to be known as getting your teeth cleaned. "Cleaning" still applies, but for the vast majority of dental patients, cleaning the teeth is just one of the many services performed by the RDH. Generally, the services provided by the majority of hygienists will fall into one of three categories. Some hygienists will do more, but all should provide evaluation, education, and hygiene therapy.

Evaluation

The RDH will use the following means in order to evaluate the health of your mouth:

- [ ] An examination for signs and symptoms (such as abscesses, cysts, and signs of cancer) of diseases other than those of the gums and teeth. Your hygienist will do this at every recall appointment and will have the dentist confirm her findings.
- [ ] Measurement and charting of the gum pockets
- [ ] Checking teeth for mobility
- [ ] X rays, when necessary
- [ ] Updating your health history at each recall visit. This is important, especially if you are taking any medication that could affect the condition of your soft tissues.
- [ ] Assessment of your overall dental health

Education

- [ ] The hygienist is a source of vital information concerning all areas of prevention. She'll not only support and guide you during your healing period but will also customize your oral hygiene program to suit your individual needs. She'll tell you about the kinds of tools you need, plus how, when, and where to use them.
- [ ] The hygienist may also provide you with valuable nutritional counseling. She isn't required to provide this service, but it's worth finding out if your hygienist does. Some hygienists are very interested in the nutritional aspect of dental prevention, and yours may be one who is.
- [ ] Your hygienist will design your personalized recall program.

Hygiene Therapy

When the hygienist gets down to the business of hygiene therapy, the procedure will consist of most of the following steps:

- [ ] Plaque and calculus (tartar) removal

- ☐ Debridement (fancy name for removal) of infected gum tissue. One day you should ask her if she's going to debride your diseased gums—then watch the look on her face.

- ☐ Application of pit and fissure sealants

- ☐ Topical fluoride treatment

- ☐ Teeth desensitization before cleaning

- ☐ Cleaning and polishing

- ☐ Monitoring your recall program

- ☐ Expanded periodontal therapy. Most advanced periodontal disease will require some treatment by the dentist or the periodontist, but hygienists are qualified to handle the disease until it reaches a certain severity. She'll tell you where that line is, and with her help you may not have to cross it.

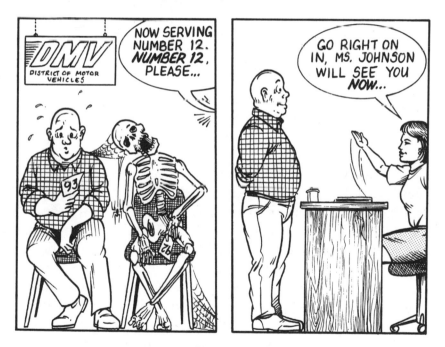

Her hygiene program will be designed with a holistic approach to your oral health. This means you should always be treated like a real, living person and not like just another mouth or a number. So if you were under the impression that all a hygienist does is clean and polish teeth, I can only ask you where you found cleaning and polishing on the previous three lists. Right, close to the bottom, after fourteen other things. In case you haven't already acknowledged it, your RDH is much more than a tooth cleaner.

YOUR ROLE

It will be almost impossible for your RDH to successfully perform her role unless you are willing to perform yours. Your hygienist knows that there's a vast difference in the oral health of those who get involved and those who don't. During her career, the typical RDH deals with thousands of different mouths as well as the personalities and attitudes that go with them. Yet, as different as all her patients are, most have three things in common:

☐ They are not as well informed as you will be.

☐ They are not nearly as motivated as you will be.

☐ They do not appreciate or fully understand how to utilize her help and support—not nearly as much as you soon will.

The fact that you will soon be well informed, motivated, and appreciative is good news for both you and your RDH. Although active hygiene therapy consumes most of the time she spends with you, she nevertheless does her best to provide you with as much preventive information as she can. Most hygienists have developed their own unique and creative approaches toward teaching dental prevention to their patients. But this already difficult task is made even more difficult when the patient lacks a basic understanding of prevention and is not self-motivated. The bottom line is that the success or failure of your oral hygiene program ultimately will be determined by your desire, your knowledge and understanding, your commitment, your attitude, and your willingness to work with her and the rest of the dental team. Results are what you are looking for. If you do your part and let your hygienist do hers, you'll get those results. Remember, you have a responsibility here, and once you know the rules, you can no longer blame the hygienist or the dentist for what you don't do. Think about that for a few moments (you could probably use a little break from reading).

The Importance of Asking Questions

Among the many valuable services offered by the RDH, one of the most important is her ability to provide you with answers to your questions. But she can't answer them if you don't ask them. So if you don't understand something, even the simplest thing, don't feel bad about asking for clarity. And don't just nod your head to indicate agreement when your brain really has not understood a word. I was a patient before I became a dentist and was as ignorant about prevention as they come. I know how tempting it is to act as if you understand everything that the hygienist is telling you just because you're too embarrassed to ask her to explain. *Believe me, few people actually know much about this subject, so you should never, ever feel that you're the only one who doesn't understand.*

Your RDH will be excited when she realizes that she actually has a patient who cares enough to learn. Wanna bet she'll love hearing and answering your questions? No! I wouldn't bet either, because I know she will. So please, don't let your ego or image get in the way of asking for help. And don't forget to jot down your questions (use the special pages in the Appendix) before your appointment so that you won't forget them when you get there.

Secrets of a Great Relationship

If you want to get the best out of your experience with your hygienist, you might want to try these suggestions:

☐ Get to know her. Take a few moments to find out about the person who'll be treating you. If you already have an RDH you should have a pretty good idea who she is. But because you're now starting from scratch, with a whole new attitude, you might want to look again.

☐ Treat your hygienist as you would wish to be treated if the roles were reversed. Be friendly and your good feeling will be returned in kind. To paraphrase an ancient saying: Your level of kindness will always attract the same level of kindness. I'll let you ponder that one for a while . . . Here's a hint. If you enter the office loaded for bear, what can you expect to be waiting for you? You got it—another bear.

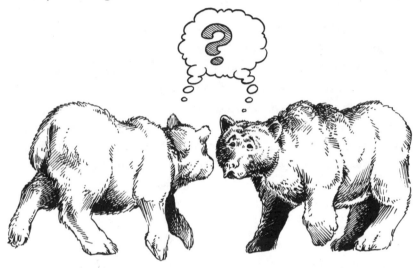

☐ Show up on time and do your hygiene homework.

☐ Tell her you're ready to do what it takes to have the healthiest mouth possible. And that you want her help. Be sincere, because she will know exactly how much you care by the end of the second appointment. If you tell someone you're a duck and you want him to believe you are, you had better be able to quack, swim, waddle, and fly.

☐ Communicate to her any fears, anxieties, or difficulties you've had with previous hygiene visits or with your existing home care program. Even if she's the same hygienist you've been seeing and you've never confided in her before, now is the time to do so. This is your chance to start over, on the right foot this time.

☐ Make a real commitment to follow the hygiene program she customizes for you. This is important, because if you think that just by reading about prevention, having a dental office support you, and having a RDH periodically clean your teeth, you will free yourself from your responsibility, you'll have to think again. For example, if you never brushed or flossed you would need a professional cleaning every few days to keep your teeth

DR. TOM'S TIPS

Most RDHs became RDHs because they care and they believe they can make a difference. Your hygienist is as much of a health professional as is your dentist or physician. You may not have been conditioned to look at her in that way, but you can take my word for it. How different is her role from that of a medical doctor who would help you save any other part of your body, like your heart or liver? She can help you keep your gums healthy and save your teeth. That makes your RDH an important and valuable asset to you, your mouth, and your health in general. Some health professionals, myself included, believe that *a person who keeps all of his teeth in a 0lifelong state of health could live five to ten years longer than the person who lives a lifetime with dental disease and eventually loses his teeth.*

This is not to say that the hygienist is more valuable to you than your general dentist or other dental specialists. They all have different roles and responsibilities, and they are all absolutely necessary to any successful preventive program. No matter how hard you may try to escape it, the necessary repair work must be done before you can ever consider your mouth restored to health. Your dentist will take care of the repair. But this book is about prevention and about making you a great patient, and in that regard, the hygienist plays the single most important role in your total preventive program.

out of serious trouble. *Your hygienist is going to care about your mouth only as much as you care about it yourself.* So tell her that you care, and show her with your *actions* that you are totally committed.

Personalities

No one is perfect, neither you nor your hygienist. Legitimate, no-fault personality problems can and do arise. If you sense a rising problem don't wait for it to get worse. Try to communicate. The patient before you could have been an insufferable jerk and you may be receiving the backlash from that difficult appointment. Or maybe your RDH is just having a bad day; we all have them. If communication doesn't clear the tension speak privately to your dentist about the problem.

If All Else Fails, or the Last Resort

If you have sincerely tried to get along with your hygienist and the relationship is still not working, even after speaking to the dentist about the situation, it may be time for a change. This could be the best thing for both of you. If it isn't working for you it probably isn't working for her either. Simply tell your RDH how you feel and begin the process of finding a new hygienist. Because most dental offices have more than one hygienist on their staff, the chances are good that you'll be able to make an in-office switch. The biggest mistake you could make would be to judge all hygienists from one experience and assume they're all the same. That attitude could inhibit your willingness to find and work with another one, which would be disastrous to your oral hygiene program.

GETTING DOWN TO BUSINESS

The RDH, as captain of the good ship SS *Hygiene,* has her own individual way of charting your course to oral health. Other hygienists might take a somewhat different course. But though there are variations on the same

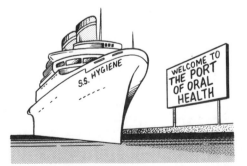

theme, all approaches will have certain things in common. What I'm presenting is the basic framework for an oral hygiene program, which your own hygienist will modify to fit your needs.

The First Appointment

The first visit with your hygienist is an important one because it will set the tone for those to come. During this appointment she'll discover what you know about dental disease and what you know about prevention. You should score pretty high on knowledge about prevention, but it will be to your advantage to let *her* decide how well you score. If you tell her you have read the chapters in *Tooth Fitness* concerning prevention, she won't need to spend a lot of time teaching you the fundamentals. She'll check your health history, examine the condition of your gums and soft tissues, record obvious decay, and pass on her evaluation to the dentist for final diagnosis. This is also the visit during which she'll chart your periodontal pockets (see Chapter 2). Because most patients know so little about this important procedure I want to tell you what it entails.

Charting the Pockets

Charting pockets is the dental term for the procedure used to measure the depth of the gingival sulcus, or gum pocket. It's a standard procedure that is accepted and used by all dentists and hygienists. Although additional methods are also used to evaluate the condition of your gums, charting the pockets is a great way for you to get a clear picture of the extent of your periodontal disease.

To measure the pocket depth, your hygienist uses a special probe that is nothing more than a round, thin, tapered ruler with a handle. Instead of inches, it is marked in millimeters (mm). She inserts the probe into the pocket

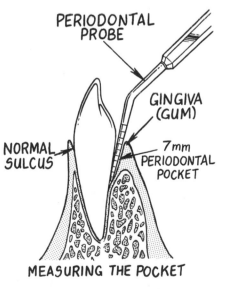

MEASURING THE POCKET

between the gum and the tooth (the instrument is smooth and the probing is painless) until the tip of the probe reaches the place where the ligament attaches to the tooth or, if the ligament has detached, until it contacts the bone. Otherwise known as the bottom of the pocket. She reads the millimeter mark at the gum line. This tells her how deep the pocket is. She continues in this way, probing the pocket in up to six places around each tooth and recording the measurements on the periodontal chart. Some hygienists are now using an electronic pocket probe that automatically reads and records the pocket depth. (Nice touch.)

Have your RDH show you the chart she uses (there are many variations on the same theme), and ask her to explain it to you. Ask her also to make a copy of your chart so you can take it home with you and keep it with your dental records.

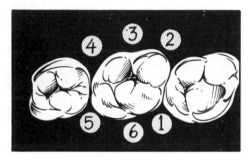

What the measurements mean   If your gums are healthy, a reading of 0 to 3 mm can be considered a healthy pocket depth. But you can have the beginnings of gingivitis (inflammation and infection of the gums) without it affecting the pockets. If the pocket depth is over 3 mm, however, you probably have not only gingivitis but also the beginnings of ligament damage and bone loss, i.e., periodontitis. Once you hit the 4 mm mark, the chances are you have full-blown periodontitis with bone loss. These readings are like a golf score: a 2 or a 3 is a lot better than a 5 or a 6. And, as the readings go higher, your hygiene program becomes more and more critical and will take more effort.

When the hygienist finishes her exam, she'll know everything she needs to know to design your oral hygiene program and direct your energy to the right areas. And if you have periodontitis, by having your pockets charted at each visit you'll have an objective method of evaluating the progress of your program. By having access to your charts at home, you can look at the numbers, compare your most recent readings to your last ones, and quickly see how well you are doing. You also won't have to rely on your memory to know which areas need the most care. Make a serious commitment to your oral hygiene program; and as your pocket depths decrease you'll know your efforts have been rewarded. That will be a good feeling.

Why they are so important I've heard that they exist, but I personally don't know of any hygienists, or dentists, who don't chart the depth of your periodontal pockets as part of the hygiene examination.

These readings are invaluable in assessing how far the periodontitis and associated bone loss has progressed within the pocket. Therefore, for the vast majority of patients, and especially for those with periodontitis, charting the depth of the pocket must be included.

Along with the pocket readings, your hygienist will also use other methods to make her final evaluation. She'll assess whatever symptoms you may have described as well as the firmness and color of your gums and whether or not there is pain, swelling, pus, tooth mobility, or bleeding. The combined results of these findings will be passed on to your dentist, and they will help him determine the severity of your periodontal disease and whether there is any permanent damage to the surrounding bone and ligaments. All these findings will determine the treatment needed and influence your hygiene program.

Pocket depth can't be determined by what the gums look like from the outside, nor can they be evaluated properly with X rays. If my hygienist were unwilling to chart my pockets, and if she didn't have an outstanding reason for not doing it (for example, in those rare cases when the gums are obviously in perfect health), I would certainly find a hygienist who would. It doesn't matter if she has been treating you for years and thinks you don't have any problem pockets—ask her to chart them anyway to ascertain that all is well. If she's been on top of it, you'll probably find that she was right, but the procedure doesn't take long and you never know. After all, it's your mouth and your money, and you two are supposed to be working together. Charting your pockets is like checking the oil in your car. If you don't do it, it could cost you an engine—or in this case, a tooth.

How Many Therapy Appointments Will You Need?

At some point, your hygienist will decide how many therapy visits your personal situation requires. She'll probably have a good idea about this after the first examination.

If your teeth and gums are in good shape most hygiene therapists will examine your mouth and clean your teeth at the same appointment. But if you have periodontitis with bone loss, lots of calculus, deep pockets, and an infection, you'll require more appointments. I speak from experience when I say that with advanced gum disease, trying to get your hygiene therapy done in one, two, or even three appointments will probably not be the best way to go . . . unless you're a masochist. Let your hygienist be the guide on this. She may need to do what is called *root planing* and *curettage*. Which means, in lay terms, that she'll have to use special tools to clean and polish the root surfaces that are now exposed. This will take more effort on her part than just cleaning and polishing the enamel. You should be prepared for, and be willing to accept, the extra time and cost this will involve. Taking a few more trips to the office and spending a few more dollars will ultimately be in your mouth's (and your pocketbook's) best interest.

If this is your situation, the time between the first and second cleanings will provide you with a great opportunity to see how much healing you can do on your own. If you diligently perform your hygiene homework, you'll soon see what a difference your efforts make when it comes time for your second cleaning procedure. You'll find it to be a lot less traumatic for your gums, yourself, and your hygienist.

The Second Appointment

Your second hygiene visit could also be called the moment-of-truth appointment. Now the hygienist will know if you meant what you said about caring and making a commitment, if you've had difficulties following her hygiene instructions, or if you're an astrological Gemini and like talking better than doing.

Usually, after you've had a chance to visit and ask her any of the questions you came up with since the first visit, she'll reexamine you, rechart your pocket depths, and finish cleaning your teeth if she needs to. The new pocket readings will allow both of you to compare the previous and present pocket depths. This is of special importance if you had pockets over 3 mm. You may not be able to actually see inside your pockets, but you sure can compare the two pocket charts. You could call them dental treasure maps because these charts will give you a wealth of information and guidance that will help you save your teeth.

With each succeeding appointment, your hygienist will continue to fine-tune your individual program. She'll point out the areas where you have produced great results, as well as areas where you haven't done so well. She'll show you where you may need to redirect your efforts.

Here's a quick quiz for you. What should you do at every visit to your hygienist? I'll give you a *big* hint: see page 339 of the Appendix. Yep, write down her comments and personalized instructions. Excellent! I am very proud of you.

If the Results Are Not Up to Snuff

If your hygiene program hasn't produced the results you are seeking, don't be discouraged. Your RDH won't be judgmental or critical as long as she knows you are sincere and are making an effort to change. She knows that you've had a lot of time in the past to form bad hygiene habits and that it sometimes takes a while to break them and form new ones. There could be a number of reasons why your efforts have not succeeded.

- ☐ It could be that you didn't understand some of the things she told you.

- ☐ Maybe you really haven't been doing your job. If not, cop to it. Talk to her about it.

- ☐ Maybe you're having a problem with dexterity and find that the brush and floss don't go where your brain tells them to go.

- ☐ Perhaps you're still having trouble establishing your new hygiene habits.

- ☐ It is also possible that you have a genetic problem or an illness that is inhibiting your body's ability to resist infection and to heal properly. (This is a very good reason to fill out your health history accurately and for the hygienist and dentist to do a thorough examination. Some health-history forms are more extensive than others. If yours doesn't list an illness or condition that you know you have, or think you may have, make sure you write it in. This isn't the time or place to hold back.)

Promise me that you'll never give up! I know if you persevere you'll soon get it all together and be able to cure this disease and stop it from ever coming back. Plus, I know that as long as you're willing to keep trying, your RDH will hang in there with you.

Additional Visits

You may require more than two visits. If so, continue getting charted and comparing the results. Remember, your efforts will succeed if you don't get discouraged. And you won't be alone. Your hygienist will continue to work with you until every last pocket of resistance has been eliminated!

If your hygiene therapy requires more than three appointments, you should have an additional follow-up evaluation two to three weeks after your final hygiene appointment. This is especially important if this was your first hygiene therapy in a while, if you haven't yet established your hygiene program, or if you have advanced periodontal disease. (If you've been a regular customer your hygienist already knows how to schedule you.) I suggest this follow-up visit so that your hygienist can give you a final evaluation and let you know how well you're doing your job. I see no reason to wait until your first recall appointment to fine-tune your hygiene program. Not all hygienists routinely schedule this type of follow-up, so you may have to request it and pay the additional fee. But in the long run, it will be well worth the time and money.

IF YOU REQUIRE PERIODONTAL SURGERY

If your dental disease is more advanced than you and your hygienist can handle, you'll need to have periodontal surgery. This that means you'll require the services of your dentist or, if it's beyond his training, the periodontist (a dentist who specializes in the treatment of advanced periodontal disease).

If you're a candidate for minor selective periodontal surgery, your hygiene efforts, along with treatment by your RDH, could very well eliminate the need. However, if you eventually end up needing surgery, your hygiene therapy program could mean that the surgery will be easier and less extensive. Because you will have already done a great deal of healing on your own, less surgery will be required. The surgery will therefore take less time. The less time it takes, the less expensive it will be. And what's more, since less diseased tissue will be involved, you'll heal faster. All these great benefits because you took responsibility for your dental health before you were sent to the periodontist.

Another bonus is that you'll already have an established oral hygiene program to fall back on after your surgery. You'll need that preventive knowledge more than ever because you'll never again have the same margin for error as someone who hasn't had periodontitis and the accompanying bone loss. When the gums heal after surgery you'll have spaces between your teeth where there were none before. That means food and plaque will have even better access to your teeth than before. *Give this a lot of thought.* You already know how difficult it is to keep your gums healthy. You've had irrefutable proof that what you tried in the past didn't work. So what do you think will happen if you don't change your previously unsuccessful hygiene program? Right . . . disaster!

If anyone, dentist or hygienist, wants to rush you to the periodontist for gum surgery before you've had a chance to at least reduce the impact of the surgery, I'd insist they provide you with a darn good reason. Legitimate emergency treatment is always the exception to this rule. I'm not suggesting that home care will always eliminate the need for periodontal surgery. But no matter how you slice it, periodontal surgery is not a barrel of fun, and you will be wise to do all you can to make it unnecessary.

THE RECALL PROGRAM

Whether it takes two visits or six, you will eventually get to the point where your hygienist will establish your personalized recall program, a schedule of hygiene appointments. This is another moment when your good work habits pay off for you in time and money. Your hygienist will decide how much time you can go between hygiene recalls based on a number of factors:

☐ Amount of gum recession and bone loss. If you have pockets over 3 mm and a lot of bone loss, it means you'll not only have to work harder at keeping them healthy but you'll also need more recall visits. Take her advice on this, even if it means ten hygiene appointments a year.

☐ Diet. Yep, what you eat will have a lot to do with how your recalls are scheduled. Most hygienists will ask you about your diet, but if yours doesn't you can try this on for size. Given the same home care and recall program, you'll need fewer cleanings the more raw and natural foods your diet contains. You will need more cleanings if your diet mainly consists of refined, soft, processed, and overcooked foods. (Take a look at Chapter 16.)

☐ Your overall attitude. She'll evaluate your stick-to-it-iveness and your willingness to stay involved with your oral hygiene program. The bottom line: the more you do, the less your RDH will have to do and the longer you can go between recall appointments.

In addition, she may take into account her own evaluation of you and your life-style. She might consider things like your personality type, your profession, your age, and certain habits that could ultimately affect the success of her treatment, such as whether you smoke, drink, or grind your teeth. Even little things, like how much you travel, can affect your recall program because taking care of your mouth when you travel is more difficult. You can be very helpful by telling her about any habit that you think is adversely affecting your oral health. She doesn't want to know in order to criticize you (what you do is up to you), but in order to help. However, she isn't Sherlock Holmes, and if you don't communicate with her you can't fault her for not figuring it out.

Farther Down the Recall Road

Over time you'll discover that the recall schedule is a living, fluid thing that is ultimately determined by you. At every recall you will be reevaluated, and one of three things could happen:

1. Your RDH will schedule less time between therapy appointments. Now why would she want to do that? You may have had so much bone loss that even the most heroic efforts at home will not prevent you from needing more frequent hygiene recalls. Or maybe you haven't gotten your hygiene program under control and can't go six months between hygiene therapies.

2. She'll keep you on the same schedule. This is a good sign. It means that there are some areas needing work, but not that many. You could be doing better, but you're still doing pretty well. Keep it up, because if you can maintain this level you can keep your teeth as long as you want. That is real empowerment. Your hygienist will continue to guide you until you get your A in home care, and when you do, she'll probably be as happy as you will be.

3. She'll let you go longer between cleanings. This is really great, and I personally salute you. It's the equivalent of getting an A in advanced intergalactic travel from Mr. Spock. You have won a battle that far too many people have lost. She may now have you back every twelve months, instead of four or six. Be proud. What you've accomplished is yours and belongs to you alone. Remember, no one followed you home. No one camped out in your bathroom and brushed your teeth for you, or flossed them, or irrigated them. No one called you to remind you to brush after every meal or before you went to bed. So please don't forget to remember to feel very good about what you have achieved. And don't forget to thank your hygienist for her support.

Another Reason for Regular Recalls

Eventually, you could go a year or more before you really need a cleaning. This will be up to you. But even after you've won your personal war against gum disease and tooth decay, there's another reason to continue regular dental visits, though it's not commonly known. Every six months you should get a soft tissue examination, both inside the mouth and in the head and neck area. This visit is especially critical if you don't regularly examine these areas yourself (see Chapter 3), or if you or anyone else in your family has a history of any of the diseases listed on page 87. As you've discovered, there are diseases other than tooth decay and gum disease that can show up in the mouth, and the few dollars and the few minutes it will take to verify freedom from them will be worthwhile both to your body and to your peace of mind. It's possible that your RDH may not feel comfortable about doing the head and neck exam. If that's the case ask your dentist to do the exam for you at each checkup.

THE COST OF HYGIENE THERAPY

The cost of routine hygiene therapy (also called *prophylaxis*) will depend on the condition of your teeth and gums, who performs the therapy, and in what part of the country you live. It's usually more expensive in cities than in rural areas. If the hygienist or the dentist has to perform root planing and curettage the cost will go up. For these two procedures, the upper and lower jaws are figuratively split down the middle, giving you four quadrants, upper left and right and lower left and right. The average fee per quadrant, in 1994, is about $150. If you have periodontal surgery the cost could be more than $500 per quadrant. Hmmm, these figures more than validate the old saying, an ounce of prevention is worth a pound of cure. Or in this case, thousands of dollars worth of treatment.

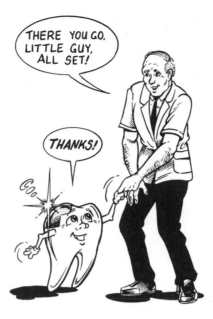

Chapter 9

Working with the Dentist

While the RDH is the most important person in your prevention process, the dentist is the key to the repair process—your tooth repair specialist. Believe me, no one else can fill this role. He's the one who will restore your teeth to health and function. You can do a lot on your own to cure and prevent dental disease, a lot more with the help of your hygienist, but until you actually get the decay repaired and restore your teeth, you'll never be able to take control over the health of your mouth. Once you get the repair taken care of, you won't have that much to do with your dentist, except for regular checkups, the replacement of broken, lost, or worn out fillings, and in emergency situations.

Oral hygiene is as important to your teeth as it is to your gums. You could find the best dentist in the universe and then spend your life's savings for the best dental repair work, but if you're not willing take care of the best work it won't last as long as mediocre repair work that is well taken care of. (This is not to excuse poor dentistry, because bad dentistry is bad . . . period, and no amount of oral hygiene will make it better. From an oral hygiene point of view, poor dentistry creates many problems and makes your home care more difficult.) How well you do your hygiene homework will have a lot to do with how long your repair work will last, be it good or poor.

As long as you need your dentist to repair the problems caused by dental disease, there are some things you should be aware of to make the best of your relationship.

THE KEYS TO MAKING YOUR COLLABORATION WORK

The keys to making your relationship work are communication and responsibility, yours and your dentist's.

Communication

I've already touched on the importance of communication in discussing your relationship with the RDH, and the same philosophy applies to your dentist. Just as with the RDH, you should never assume anything. If you want to set off on the right track you have to take the time to communicate your feelings and your needs from the beginning. This approach will save you both a lot of stress and trauma. The consultation period is an excellent time to do this, but you should be able to talk with him whenever the need arises. If he doesn't value your input or can't take the time to listen to you and respond to your needs, you should find a dentist who will.

If your dentist is a wise man—and that's the kind of man you want working for you—he'll value and appreciate your interest and involvement. He will also recognize that your concern about your dental health is as valuable to him as it is to you.

Responsibility

The other key to a successful dental experience is responsibility. The dentist has a responsibility to do everything he can for your teeth, to the very best of his ability—to be, in short, the best dentist he can be. Naturally, this is a two-sided coin, and if you want him to be the best dentist he can be, you'll have to be the best patient you can be. With the right approach on your part, it will be easy to get him on your side.

The important thing is to make it clear to him that you're not a typical patient. Like the hygienist, he sees too many typical patients. Most patients don't seem to appreciate his efforts and his importance to their dental health. Your new attitude will be like a breath of fresh air. You want him to know that not only do you have the information you need to be the best patient he's ever seen, but you also have the willingness to take on that responsibility, at home and at the dental office.

Your responsibilities are as follows:

☐ Come on time. If you must be late let the office know.

☐ If possible, don't cancel without at least a twenty-four-hour notice.

☐ Pay your bills on time. Remember, you should only accept a treatment plan that you can realistically afford.

☐ Follow the instructions of the dentist and the RDH.

☐ Be willing to trust. This means you'll trust your dentist to offer the best treatment for your unique oral situation, as long as this trust is warranted by his actions.

In return for assuming your responsibility, here's what you can expect from your dentist:

☐ He'll be on time. Occasionally he may be late, because he can't control every situation, and emergencies do crop up. But if lateness is habitual, talk to him about it.

☐ He'll make every effort to eliminate the pain and discomfort of your dental experience. Tell him, ahead of time, about any fears or anxieties you may have.

☐ He'll be responsive to your needs, listen to you, and answer all your questions.

☐ He'll be honest with you at all times.

☐ He'll treat you like a human being.

All dentists are held accountable to uphold certain standards. They must be licensed by the state and must take continuing education courses to maintain their license. A dentist who is a member of the American Dental Association (ADA) will be subject to a review of his peers if a patient lodges a complaint against him. A dentist who is not an ADA member is not subject to such a review, but not being a member in no way means he would not be an excellent dentist. But regardless of his membership, *you are ultimately the only one who can really hold him accountable*. No one is better suited to regulate him than you. Once he realizes that you know what is expected of him and will accept only the best, he will truly be working for you.

I believe that any dentist who takes pride in his practice and his ability will love seeing a patient who understands the basics of prevention. He'll realize that the work he does for you will be taken care of, that he'll be appreciated for his extra efforts, and that a happy person will soon be spreading his good reputation by word-of-mouth.

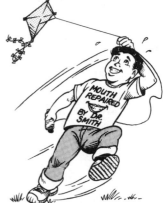

THE TREATMENT PLAN

When you feel confident that you've found a dentist who is right for you, it's time to deal with the practical side of dental repair. To make sure you get the best treatment plan possible, tell the dentist, during your initial visit, that you want the same treatment plan he would use if he were treating his own mouth instead of yours. After the examination, X rays, and hygiene therapy, you'll have a consultation with the dentist and he'll present you with one or more treatment plans. Using the information he has gleaned from his exam, the X rays, and the hygienist, he will have determined the best way to restore your mouth to health and proper function. The presentation of the treatment plan is one of the most important consultations you will ever have with the dentist.

When he submits your treatment plan(s), you must be 200 percent clear about what will be done, why it will be done, how it will be scheduled, how much it will cost, and how you will pay for it. Most dentists operate within a very tight and busy schedule, and if they're not requested to explain everything they might not take the time to do so. In our world, time is money. Of course, you may have already established such a trusting relationship with your dentist that you don't need to have everything explained in minute detail. To make the right decision you don't have to know about dental equipment, the best way to prepare a dental restoration, and all the other stuff a dentist learns in school.

But you do need to know what he's going to do to your teeth and why. This begins when he presents possible treatment plans. It's up to you, working with your dentist, to choose the best one. Your ultimate decision will be based on your age, the condition of your gums and bone, your ability to take care of your mouth, your financial situation, and aesthetic considerations. Every situation is different, and what's good for the goose is *not* always good for the gander.

You don't want him to present a treatment plan based on what he thinks you can afford. It is not in your best interest to make such an important decision on the basis of cost rather than quality. If you're willing to do your preventive homework you'll be financially and functionally better off if you spend the extra money to have your dental work done right the first time. If you don't choose the best treatment plan you'll end up spending more money in the long run because you'll be continually replacing fillings. Thus, if you have a tooth that can be filled by an amalgam filling, but would eventually have to be replaced by a crown, you would be better off going for the crown, even though it costs more now, and saving the added cost of the amalgam filling.

Once your dentist knows you are totally devoted to taking care of your mouth, he may be willing to offer you a payment plan that would allow you to get the best quality treatment now. Many dentists give a discount if you pay in cash, so ask the receptionist if he does.

On the other hand, if you're not willing to take care of your mouth the cheapest dental work is the way to go—it will eventually fail, but there's no sense spending money on quality, long-lasting fillings if you're not going to take care of your mouth. It's frustrating for the conscientious dentist to try to explain to you that his work failed because of your poor oral hygiene.

When comparing your treatment options, ask the dentist how long the restorative work proposed with each treatment plan can be expected to last. Not all restorations last the same length of time.

This information will be extremely important when it comes to making your final decision. If a less expensive restoration is estimated to last five years and a more expensive one to last ten years, it's probably better in the long run to get the one that lasts longer. As you well know, prices always seem to go up, not down. So, if the less expensive one has to be replaced in five years it will end up being more expensive than the ten-year plan.

My twenty years of experience dealing with dental patients have proven to me that unless patients know and appreciate the value of their teeth, they'll always be able to justify why they shouldn't spend money on them. That's too bad. Until you've lost them, you'll never know how valuable your natural teeth are. So make sure you get the best treatment plan available, and if you can't afford the best, get the best you can afford. Believe me, it's not my intention to promote more business for the dentist. In fact, it's just the opposite—I don't want you to spend a nickel more than you have to. But I'd be letting you down if I didn't make it clear that it's in your own best interests to have the highest-quality treatment possible. But make sure you take care of the work you have done. If you do, you'll be one happy dental patient.

SPECIAL CONSIDERATIONS

Although you don't need to get into the technicalities of how to fill teeth or what goes into making a bridge, there are a few things you should know about dentistry. Having some basic knowledge in these areas will help you understand why certain procedures must be done and will save the dentist from having to explain them to you.

Decay

All decay must be removed and the tooth repaired. Every day you postpone treatment will end up costing you more money, more time, and more of your tooth. It would be great if filling a tooth meant you only had to remove the decayed part.Unfortunately, that's not always the case. The decay, once it gets into the dentin, often spreads out in all directions. Many times the decay will undermine the enamel that supports the dentin, and the enamel above the dentin will have to be removed. If it isn't, the enamel will collapse. The filling material needs the support of the enamel and the dentin to make the filling stay in place and to withstand the forces exerted upon it from chewing. If your dentist says you have a little decay, but he has to remove a lot of the tooth in order to place the restoration, you'll know why. If the decay extends to the side of a tooth he will need to remove enough tooth structure to allow him to place the margins of the filling into areas that can be easily cleaned. This is important to prevent new decay at the vulnerable area where the tooth meets the filling.

Missing Teeth

If you want to restore your mouth to health and function, missing teeth must be replaced. (There are some exceptions, like wisdom teeth.) If you don't have them replaced you'll be creating many problems. These range from a loss of chewing function, a bad bite, and possibly temporomandibular joint (TMJ) problems, to the increased probability of decay and periodontal disease. Many things have a good news–bad news side to it, but there's no good news when it comes to missing teeth. The longer you wait to have teeth replaced, the more money it will cost you. Your dentist will provide you with all the options regarding the best and longest-lasting way to replace them, but whether you need bridges, partial dentures, full dentures, or implants, it's in the best interest of your mouth, your digestive system, and your general health to have a full set of teeth, real or false. (See Chapter 15, "Dentures and Implants.")

Tooth Extraction

If your dentist insists on extracting a tooth (or teeth), make sure you speak to him first and explore all the options available to save it. He may be suggesting this only because he assumes you won't pay to have it repaired. Having a tooth extracted may seem less expensive in the short run, but it definitely will not be in the long run.

Many teeth can be saved with proper treatment, repair, and hygiene. However, there are those that are too far gone to save, no matter what you and your dentist do. Most of the teeth that fall into the cannot-be-saved category are those which have fallen prey to periodontal disease so advanced that there's no longer enough bone surrounding the tooth to support it. In some cases, these teeth may be saved for a few years—as long as they're not needed to support a bridge or a partial. Teeth with fractured roots also usually fall into the cannot-be-saved category. If your dentist decides that a tooth will not support a bridge for any reasonable length of time, he may recommend extraction.

I suggest you tell him that you want to save every tooth you can, and if it's a borderline situation tell him you want to see if you can keep it healthy before he makes a final decision. Always ask him to explain why he feels a tooth can't be saved, and if, after his explanation, you still have doubts, ask him to refer you to a periodontist for a second opinion. The main thing is to make sure your dentist is not recommending a tooth extraction just because he thinks you won't take care of your teeth in the future or won't pay to have it repaired. It's up to you to let him know that you're now a responsible patient and to convince him that you're willing to do whatever it takes to save your teeth.

Fractures

Whenever part of a tooth has broken off, it will always have to be restored, even if the tooth doesn't hurt. The exception is if it's a small chip that can be smoothed.

If you fracture a cusp the function it normally provides in grinding and chewing your food is lost. A fractured tooth can also lead to a bite problem. If it is serious enough, goes on long enough, and the teeth shift their position, you could eventually create TMJ trouble.

Lost Fillings

If you've lost a filling you won't die. You will still be able to eat many foods, talk, and do just about everything else you could do before you lost it. That's the good news. The bad news is that if you don't have it replaced you will lose much, or all, of that tooth's chewing function, along with the function of the tooth above or below it. Thus, you will have lost the use of two teeth. You will have also increased the chances of that tooth becoming decayed (there won't be any enamel to protect it), as well as dramatically increased its chances of fracturing. Losing one tooth can have a domino effect and could eventually lead to the loss of its former partner.

X rays

Ah, to x-ray or not to x-ray. Everyone has an opinion about this, and I do too. X rays are a great preventive tool when used correctly. Most beginning decay can't be seen by the naked eye, especially in the contact areas, under fillings, and below the gum line. As the decay progresses, however, the dentist can often see it. But once it's invaded the dentin, he can't determine how far it's progressed. If it were not for X rays the dentist wouldn't know the extent of the decay before he drilled, nor could he tell you ahead of time the type of restoration you'd need. In some cases, if it weren't for X rays, your first warning of the danger you're in would be pain.

There are three types of X rays. The first is the *full-mouth set* of X rays, where every tooth and all of the roots are x-rayed. If you have all your teeth it will normally take eighteen X rays to do the job. The second type is the *bitewing X ray*, where only the top parts of the back teeth are x-rayed. This type of X ray is used to reveal decay between the teeth and below the gum line. The third type is called the *periapical X ray*. It is used to check for problems at the tips of the roots. It also gives a good picture of the bone that surrounds the teeth and is a critically important diagnostic tool for evaluating bone loss. It is absolutely necessary in root canal treatment.

If you change dentists you should always have your X rays, or a copy of them, sent to your new dentist. If they're up-to-date, you won't have to have new X rays taken.

You should always have a full-

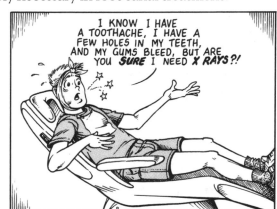

I KNOW I HAVE A TOOTHACHE, I HAVE A FEW HOLES IN MY TEETH, AND MY GUMS BLEED, BUT ARE YOU *SURE* I NEED *X RAYS*?!

mouth set of X rays if you fall into any of the following categories:

- ☐ You have not had a dental examination, treatment, or a full-mouth set taken in at least three years.

- ☐ You have not taken care of your teeth and gums and you have obvious signs of periodontal disease and decay.

☐ You are at least sixteen and have never had a full-mouth set taken.

Once you have your hygiene trip together and have had your teeth repaired, you should have bitewing X rays taken every twelve to eighteen months. If no decay shows up for three years, you can stretch that interval to every two years, or even longer. Your dentist will guide you here. Other than these routine checks, you don't need to have X rays taken unless you have an emergency or a symptom that would warrant an X ray—a painful or sensitive tooth, an incoming wisdom tooth that is giving you trouble, or any swelling or tenderness around the root of a tooth.

Children and X rays In most cases there's no need to x-ray a child's teeth before the age of five. Even then, I wouldn't recommend them unless they are obviously needed to prepare for orthodontic treatment or to diagnose areas of rampant decay. If your child has been taking good care of her mouth she should only need bitewings from the age of five to sixteen. These are my suggestions; your dentist may find good reason to x-ray your child sooner. If he does, make sure he clearly explains his reasons.

Protecting yourself from X rays Today's X ray machines are vastly superior to those of the past and deliver only the amount of X rays needed to develop the film (which is more sensitive). Unless you have a job that exposes you to X rays or you are pregnant, there's really no reason to be concerned about routine dental X rays. Every office I know of uses protective lead shields on the patient when taking X rays. If the staff forgets to do this, be sure to remind them. Today they use one to protect your body and one to protect your throat because the thyroid gland is especially vulnerable to X rays.

Reading X rays It isn't necessary for you to become a dentist or an X ray technician in order to be a good patient, so I won't teach you how to read X rays. What I do suggest is that you ask your dentist to show you X rays of both your decayed and your healthy teeth so that you can see the difference. He will point out existing fillings, bone loss, abscessed teeth, or anything else you should know about. Reading X rays takes skill and experience, so you'll have to trust your dentist.

Some dentists use the *panograph* X *ray* procedure and computer-generated X rays. The panograph is a continuous X ray scan taken of both jaws. The film is placed outside the body, and it is easier to take than periapical and bitewing X rays. In my opinion, it's not as valuable for diagnosing all types of decay and gum disease as are traditional X rays, although it is used to do so. Its greatest value lies in its ability to evaluate serious oral-facial abnormalities that involve more than just the teeth. The new technology of computer-generated X rays requires a very expensive machine, but the radiation exposure you receive is very small, equivalent to one regular X ray. Both of these techniques are being used more and more and can be very valuable. But if your dentist wants to do a panograph on you, I suggest you make sure he fully explains why.

Intraoral Camera

This device is one of the newest additions to dental diagnosis and patient education. In essence, it's like having a TV camera take pictures inside your mouth. It can do periodontal charting, take digital X rays, assist with treatment planning, and do cosmetic imaging. The thing I like about it is that it takes you inside your mouth, in color, and allows you to see things you may never have seen before. These cameras are expensive and not every dentist has one. If your dentist doesn't own one, it in no way means he can't do his job as well as one who does.

SECOND OPINIONS

If you've found a good dentist, chances are you won't often need to seek a second opinion. Nevertheless, situations do arise when one is warranted.

When to Seek a Second Opinion

You should consider obtaining a second opinion when you're faced with a complicated and costly procedure and have serious doubts about whether you need it; when work needs to be done that can also be performed by a specialist and you're unsure of your dentist's qualifications to perform it; when you don't have trust in your dentist; or when you have a rare condition with which your dentist is not familiar.

How to Evaluate a Second Opinion

Getting a second opinion does not always guarantee that it will resolve your dilemma. What if one dentist tells you one thing and the other tells you something different? Not being a dentist yourself, you may not find it easy to make a decision. But I can give you some guidelines to follow:

☐ If you have to make a choice between a general dentist's opinion and a dental specialist's, choose that of the specialist.

☐ If the potential treatment involves anything other than simple fillings, crowns, bridges, or uncomplicated dentures, and the choice is between two general dentists, choose the one with the most experience.

☐ If your choice is between what is cheapest and what is best, and you can afford it, take the best.

☐ When all has been said, but not yet done, choose the dentist who stresses prevention, who is willing to answer all of your questions and explain each procedure in question—and whom you trust the most.

There will be times when the only way to make a decision will be to obtain a third opinion—if the treatment you're considering involves a lot of money, is an uncommon procedure, or is extraordinarily complicated.

PART THREE

The Rest of the Story:
Read It When You Need It

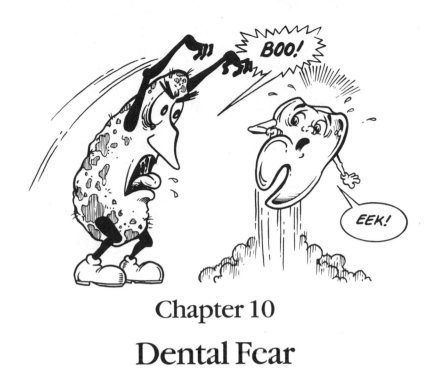

Chapter 10

Dental Fear

The American Dental Association estimates that half the people in the United States have some fear of dentistry. Other sources estimate that as many as 40 million people are so afraid of the dental experience that they avoid treatment altogether. Because of their fear they risk losing their teeth rather than seek dental treatment.

Whatever you want to call it—fear, anxiety, worry, or apprehension—you pay for it in many ways. For one, you suffer the psychological trauma of the fear. Fear places stress on your body, and when it's combined with the stress of dental disease your health will be severely undermined. Your phobia can also cost you a great deal of money because if it keeps you from the dentist until you eventually need to have all of your teeth extracted, you'll end up with the expense of dentures. It will affect your social life and your self-esteem, too, because dental disease causes unsightly tooth loss, ruins your smile, and contributes to bad breath. No matter how you look at it, you suffer more from not dealing with your fear than you ever would from treating your dental disease.

Fear, according to the dictionary, is a strong and unpleasant emotion caused by anticipation of danger. In other words, people with dental fear perceive something dangerous in the dental experience. They expect something bad to happen to them. Most dental phobias stem from a painful and traumatic experience of the past that has left a seemingly indelible impression. You may have had this experience when you were five, or you may have had it last week. If you're so anxious about going to the dentist that it delays—or prevents—you from seeking regular treatment, this could be the most important chapter in the book.

COMMON REASONS FOR DENTAL PHOBIA

Few people are afraid of the entire dental experience. Generally they have a fear of one or more aspects of the dental visit. When the particular fear has been isolated it can be dealt with. The following is a list of the most common dental phobias:

- ☐ Fear of the dentist
- ☐ Fear of the unknown
- ☐ Fear of pain
- ☐ Fear of the injection (shot)
- ☐ Fear of the equipment
- ☐ Fear of the drill (hand piece)
- ☐ Fear of confinement
- ☐ Fear of gagging
- ☐ Fear of being embarrassed
- ☐ Fear of the cost

Is your particular fear on the list? It's one thing to know what it is and another to know what you can do about it. So let's look at ways to help you overcome your phobia.

SOME SPECIFIC FEARS AND REMEDIES

Fear of the Dentist

Fear of the dentist is the easiest fear to resolve, and it's also the key to dealing with all the others. First, if you're still seeing a dentist who's not responsive to your fears and anxieties, or is actually the cause of your phobia, don't go back to him—ever. Second, never stop seeking dental treatment because you've had a bad experience. Don't judge the rest of the apples by one bad one. All dentists aren't the same. Third, look for a new dentist and don't stop until you find one who responds to your needs. Trust me, there are excellent dentists out there, who do care, and who are willing and trained to deal with every aspect of dental fear. (If you haven't read it already, you can refer to Chapter 6 to help you find a good dentist.)

When you begin your search for an understanding dentist you should start with the receptionist. Ask her if her employer is caring and responsive to the concerns of the fearful dental patient. Tell her what things make you nervous, and ask her to make a note of them on your personal dental chart. When you arrive for your first visit with the dentist, repeat your concerns to him. Then, give your new dentist a chance. He's not the same one that caused your fear, and if you give him a chance he'll help you deal with it.

Fear of the Unknown

Since all fear is anxiety about the unknown, something that hasn't happened yet, you could say that fear is actually a creation of the imagination. And often our imaginations work overtime when it comes to painting fearful pictures. Your imagination may get help from those horror stories told to you by family, friends, or strangers. Or perhaps you've seen dentists portrayed in negative ways in cartoons, by comedians, in books, or in film. The best way to deal with an overactive imagination is to make sure the dentist explains absolutely everything—what he'll be doing to you, and why. You should know exactly what to expect. This is especially important if your treatment involves something you've never experienced before. Understanding the reality of the procedure dispels what the imagination has created and turns the unknown into the known.

Fear of Pain

This is a biggie, it's true—but it can be dealt with. The two most effective ways to deal with a fear of pain are, first, to find a caring dentist and, second, to make sure that you are fully numbed before any procedure begins and that you remain numb throughout it.

This means that if you feel pain (and I don't mean pressure on your lip, cheek, or tongue), call a halt and ask for more anesthetic. Don't buy into the "This will only hurt a little bit, you don't need a shot" or "I'm almost finished, no need to give you another shot" business. It's your pain, not the dentist's. A good dentist will always be responsive to your feelings and your needs.

Fear of the Injection (Shot)

The injection of yesterday isn't the injection of today. The needles used today are so small and so sharp that you'd have to *try* to give a painful shot. Some dentists even use a pressure injection device where no needle is used.

All good dentists are aware of the tricks that can make a shot painless. Usually they will first apply a topical anesthetic on the area to be injected in order to numb the skin. They'll heat the local anesthetic to body temperature so that the tissue around the injection site won't react to the difference in temperature. A good injection will be a slow injection. The dentist will slowly inject a small amount of anesthetic around the nerves, numbing the area, and then inject the remaining solution, slowly in order not to bruise the delicate tissues. This technique reduces the soreness usually caused by a rapid injection, where the solution is deposited with a great deal of pressure.

There are various "diverter techniques" (I talk about them a little later on) you can practice to keep your attention away from the shot. Breathing nitrous oxide (laughing gas) prior to the shot can also be helpful in reducing anxiety. Give your dentist a chance to use all the pain-avoiding procedures at his disposal. But if he doesn't, and the injections still hurt, remind him of some of these pain-relieving options. If there's still no response, find a dentist who will respond.

Fear of the Equipment

Many traumatic experiences are directly related to outdated equipment and techniques. If your concept of dental treatment is based on techniques from the dinosaur age, you're in for a big surprise. The advances in dental technology have been phenomenal. The technology of today is not only a thousand times better than that of thirty years ago—it's a hundred times better than only ten years ago. If your fear is the result of a miserable experience that you had many years ago, you owe it to yourself and your mouth to give modern dentistry a chance.

Fear of the Drill (Hand Piece)

Most people aren't afraid of the hand piece itself but of the pain they associate with the drilling. They may even become anxious just at the sound of the drill. If this is the case with you, bring a cassette player and your favorite tape (with earphones, of course). Or use ear plugs.

The drilling only causes pain if you're not sufficiently anesthetized (numbed). Before the procedure begins, establish with your dentist, and his assistant, a hand signal that you can use to stop the procedure at any time. If you feel any pain during the drilling, use the signal and ask for another shot. Once you know that you have this control, you'll be more able to relax and get comfortably through the procedure.

Fear of Confinement

Some people experience a fear of confinement when in the dental chair. Others fear not being in control. Of course, these aren't really dental problems per se, and the best approach is probably to consult a psychotherapist. But if you let your dentist know that you have these fears there are ways he can cooperate to help you minimize them. He can schedule shorter appointments, and when you feel anxiety coming on, he can stop the procedure so you can get up and walk around.

Fear of Gagging

Gagging is most commonly seen when a full-mouth impression is taken, especially of the upper jaw and teeth. Let your dentist know if you've had a problem with gagging because there are certain things he can do to minimize the gagging reflex. The techniques I've found most effective are reducing the amount of impression material used, using the smallest impression tray possible, and using a topical anesthetic or an anesthetic gargle to numb the back of the mouth.

Fear of Being Embarrassed

A surprising number of people are afraid of being embarrassed in the dental office. Usually they haven't been to the dentist for many years and have not taken care of their mouths. They think the dentist or hygienist will be upset or disgusted, or think less of them. Don't buy into that attitude—it just isn't true. A caring dentist (and that's who you want) will be happy that you had the courage to walk in the door. I applaud anyone who takes that first step toward overcoming dental disease, and I know he will, too.

Fear of the Cost

A majority of people recently surveyed said that they were more afraid of how much their dental treatment would cost than of any other part of their dental experience. I don't blame them for their concerns. But cost is no reason not to have the damage repaired, even if you have to borrow the money. I say this because your health is at stake and because the repair work you need to have done will always be less costly today than later on. Pay me now, or pay me a lot more tomorrow.

Other Fears

You may have other, less common but nevertheless real fears. Whatever they may be, the best way to deal with them is to let your dentist know what they are. If he doesn't know, he can't help; but if he does know, he can be a great source of support.

OTHER METHODS OF DEALING WITH FEAR AND STRESS

In the previous section, I isolated some of the specific fears people experience and suggested some specific remedies. Now let's look at some other beneficial methods and techniques that are effective for a whole range of dental fears.

☐ *Turning your fear into motivation* Many unwilling dental patients have two opposing fears: the fear of the dental experience and the fear of losing their teeth. *Think about that.* If you were going to put any energy into fear, wouldn't it make more sense to put it into the fear of losing your teeth and to use it to overcome the fear of the dental experience? If you don't go to

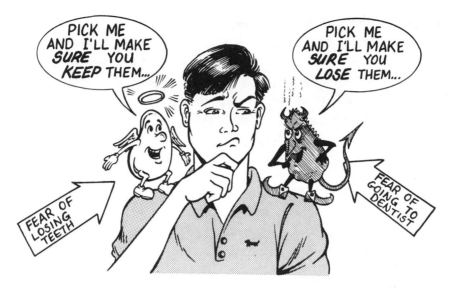

the dentist now, you'll end up going later anyway—for emergency visits and tooth extractions. At least until you end up losing all your teeth. In the long run, you can't avoid going to the dentist. Given that fact, try my logic on for size: If you bundle up your courage and have your teeth and gums treated and repaired, it may take six or seven visits to the dentist. On the other hand, if you wait until emergencies force you to go, and eventually have all your teeth extracted, you could easily total thirty or forty visits (and end up spending much more money). I'll let you decide . . .

☐ *Phobia centers* Most fearful dental patients will be able to overcome their fears by finding a caring and supportive dentist and following the specific suggestions offered in this chapter. But for some of you, professional help will be the way to go if you want to save your teeth. I know you think your fear is real and justified and that it will last forever, but you really can get help. So if it seems impossible to deal with on your own, or with your dentist's help, seek out a fear center. You'll receive individual help from specialists who are trained to help people deal with their particular fears. To find the phobia center nearest you, call the local dental association, the nearest dental school, or your hospital for a referral. *The Tooth Fitness Digest* will keep you updated about new ways to deal with dental fear.

☐ *Psychotherapy* Psychologists and psychotherapists are well trained to deal with fear of all kinds, including dental, and will be a great help. One of the methods they may use is hypnosis. If you've been skeptical about hypnosis, but nothing else you've tried has helped, you owe it to your oral health to try this approach. If you were dying of thirst in the desert, I don't think you'd care who gave you the water that saves your life.

Today it seems that everyone knows at least one person who is seeing a therapist. If you know a person who is seeing one, that's the best place to start. If you can't get a referral this way, look in the yellow pages, under Psychologists, or call the state or local psychology association and ask for the name of a therapist in your area who specializes in treating the fearful patient.

☐ *Meditation* I know some people who took up meditation just to help them deal with their dental fears (and found that it also helped them deal with the rest of life's problems). In a broad sense meditation acts as a mind diverter. If you do it correctly you can focus your attention away from the dental event at hand. It's also very relaxing and can be used to calm yourself while in the waiting room. There are many books on how to meditate, but the best I've found is *How to Meditate* by John Novak. (It's published by Crystal Clarity, and you can order it by calling 800-424-1055.)

ALLEVIATING STRESS DURING THE VISIT

Not many people will confuse going to the dentist with a picnic. But even if it isn't the most enjoyable way to spend your time, there are some things that you can do to make it far better than it's been in the past. These suggestions aren't just for those of you who are anxious or afraid, but for anyone who wants to make their dental journey a better one, both physically and emotionally.

☐ Schedule your visit, if possible, before noon. Your nerves are better, you usually have more energy, and according to some studies, you're better able to deal with stress in the morning. If you're going to have a long appointment, schedule it so you'll be able to go home and rest after it's over.

☐ Take an aspirin or two before you get worked on (one-half to one hour prior). This is a great way to help alleviate the little pains and discomforts that often accompany even the most routine dental visit. Pain relievers are actually more effective at *preventing* pain than they are at *relieving* it. If you knew you were going to get a headache, two aspirins taken before would work much better than two aspirins taken after the pain had already taken hold. If you plan to follow this advice, be sure to inform your dentist beforehand. He may have a reason why you shouldn't, and he may also tell you if there's a more effective pain reliever available to you.

☐ Bring a book with you, one you really enjoy. It'll help pass the time in the waiting room, and you may even get a chance to read it while in the dental chair.

☐ Many dental offices offer stereo earphones. However, I suggest you bring your own setup, for two reasons: first, you can have complete control over what you listen to, and second, it's easier for the dentist to work on you if the cords from his stereo are not in the way.

☐ Talk to your dentist and his assistant before any procedure gets going and work out a stop signal. You can use it to let them know if you're feeling pain or if you want them to stop for any other reason. The most popular signal is raising a hand. The dental assistant is trained to watch for your signal, and when you use it the dentist will stop and you'll have a chance to express your feelings. Don't wait until the procedure is finished to let him know it hurt. If you tough it out you'll not only have to endure the pain but will end up blaming him for causing it. This isn't fair to the dentist— he doesn't have a crystal ball.

☐ Watch your thoughts. When you catch them creating anxiety, focus on your breathing. Take a few slow, deep breaths, and focus your attention on following each breath, in and out. If you wander, come back and start over. Once you master this technique you'll find it very calming. You can also shift your thoughts to other, more pleasant things, such as an exotic dish you're going to prepare, or a sunrise walk on the beach, or your next vacation in Hawaii. Control your thoughts; don't let them control you.

☐ Practice "attention diverters." The purpose of these techniques is to divert your attention from where you don't want it—in this case, the dental work being done. The reason they work is that it's almost impossible for the mind to focus on more than one thing at a time. Therefore, if you put your attention on something else, your mind can't also focus on the work being done to you.

One technique is to raise your foot or your arm a few inches off the dental chair and hold it there. Not only does this take some physical effort but it also demands a lot of mental attention. When your leg gets tired, fight the urge to lower it—you'll find you're focusing more on your leg than on whatever is going on in your mouth. But be sure and stop before your entire body begins to vibrate, because it's no fun for the dentist to work on a vibrating patient. Give it a rest and begin again, as needed.

Another "diverter" you can use is to contract and then relax your muscles. Start with your right foot (contract, and then relax) move to the calf (contract, relax), then the thigh, then your right hand, forearm, and upper arm. Move to your left upper arm and proceed in the same fashion down to your left foot. Begin again. This is not only a diverter but it's also very relaxing.

These diverter techniques are great when you find you're becoming anxious about something that you associate with pain—a shot, drilling, X rays, the taking of impressions. Ask your dental assistant if she knows any other diverter techniques you can try. She'll tell you which ones work the best.

☐ During a procedure, whenever there's a break in the action, do whatever stretching and massage techniques you can fit in. You might be able to do neck rolls, and opening, closing, and rotating your lower jaw in a circular motion. If there's time you might be able to stand up and stretch. Do this at every opportunity. The most effective areas to massage are around the TMJ (found just in front of the ear lobe), the muscles of mastication (put your fingertips on the area between your cheekbone and ear lobe; open and close and you'll feel these muscles), and on your neck and shoulders.

☐ There are numerous drugs that the dentist can give you before a treatment to help alleviate your anxiety. He'll know which is the best one for your situation, but if you don't tell him of your fears he may not suggest them to you.

☐ If you find that, no matter what you do, you can't overcome your fears to the degree that will allow you to have the necessary repair work done, you can opt for general anesthesia. It's more expensive, but it's a sure-fire way to eliminate that oppressive fear. All general anesthesia involves a risk, so if this is the way you decide to go make sure you select a dentist who specializes in this and always check his credentials and references. Your dentist, or the local dental association, will know which dentists are skilled in this procedure.

ALLEVIATING STRESS AFTER THE VISIT

Every visit to the dentist or hygienist can be divided into three stages: before you arrive, while you are there, and after you leave. I have spoken about what you can do to help the "before" and the "during." Now I'll suggest ways to make the "after" better.

☐ If you can afford it, schedule a professional massage after a long dental visit. This is such a great way to unwind. If you can't get someone else to massage you, at least massage yourself. Massage the muscles around the TMJ, the facial muscles generally, and especially your neck and shoulders.

☐ A nice hot bath can do wonders to help you relax after a long dental visit.

☐ After some procedures the dentist may provide you with pain pills. The fearful patient should always take advantage of this. Take them as soon after the visit as possible, but always according to his specific instructions. If someone is driving you home, you can take them at the dental office. If not, wait until you get home. If you take the pain reliever soon as possible, it could begin to take effect about the time the shot wears off. It will provide relief from postoperative pain and from the aches and tension of sitting in one place for a long period with your mouth open. Dentists often recommend aspirin or Motrin because they not only relieve pain but are also effective anti-inflammatory agents.

☐ Never eat anything until the shot has completely worn off, especially if your tongue has been numbed. You won't know where it is and you could easily bite it. This is a fairly common side effect, so pay attention and be gentle.

☐ Being numb is admittedly a strange sensation. You lose awareness of where your lip is located, and it might feel as if it's swollen, but it isn't. Some people dislike this feeling so much that they'd rather have their dental work done without an injection. That's fine if you can go through the procedure without screaming and jumping around, but if you can't go through it in a relaxed way, it'll be very difficult for the dentist to work on you. No dentist I know enjoys working on a patient he knows is in pain.

☐ The tingling that you experience when the shot begins to wear off indicates that the nerves are beginning to come back to life. If you don't like the sensation there are a few things you can do to make it go away faster. Move the lips, tongue, and

DR. TOM'S TIPS

Fear should no longer be a reason to lose your teeth. In recent years the dental profession has fully acknowledged the need to treat and support the millions of fearful patients who suffer from dental phobia and have evolved many new techniques to effectively deal with it.

But just think, if you had known how to take care of your mouth in the first place you would never have had any dental problems. If you didn't need any treatment you wouldn't be going through any fear about it. Simple, huh? When it comes right down to it, prevention is the most foolproof way to deal with all dental phobias.

the other muscles of the face in every conceivable way as soon as possible after your appointment. Make faces, open your mouth wide, tighten up and relax, stick your tongue out and in. This increases blood flow to the area and removes the anesthetic more rapidly. Gently massage the numb area, but be careful not to use too much pressure (since it's numb you won't be able to judge if you're being too rough). You could also try placing hot, moist packs on the tingling area. But always check with your dentist before you do any of these things because after certain procedures he may not want you to do a lot of movement.

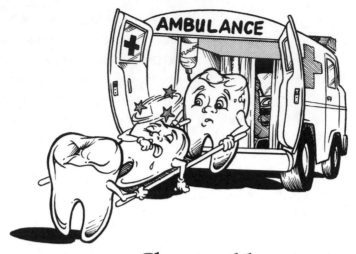

Chapter 11

Dental Emergencies

A s far as I'm concerned, you have an emergency situation as soon
as your teeth or gums have become diseased. You can either catch
it early (while it's still a little emergency), through periodic dental examinations and repair, or wait until your body's defense mechanisms
can no longer fight off the disease. Then you've got a big emergency.

An *emergency* is a condition that needs immediate attention.
If unattended, the results will be immediate and further deterioration of the affected part. What people generally don't realize is that
pain usually doesn't show up until after the damage has occurred, except in
an acute situation like an accident. You most certainly can have an
emergency with little or no pain involved. This means you can't afford to let pain be the sole indicator of a dental emergency. Millions
of people are walking around with a dental emergency because they
believe a dental emergency must always be associated with pain.

Much suffering and expense have resulted from patients not
recognizing this fact. A tooth can literally be rotting away inside—
and you may never see or feel it until it's too late. The bone that supports your teeth in the jaw can slowly be dissolving—and you may
only get hints of the destruction. When it comes to an emergency,
remember these words: *big or little, the sooner the better*.

I hope you've never had one, and never will have one, but in case you, or a family member, or a friend, ever find yourself in an emergency situation, you should know what to look for and what you can do about it at home.

SIGNS AND SYMPTOMS

Every emergency situation will have signs and symptoms that you'll be able to recognize. The following are the most common signs of a dental emergency:

- ☐ **Pain** Pain is the most obvious symptom, especially if it's severe or recurrent. But even if you only get an isolated jolt of pain that decreases or goes away after taking a pain reliever, don't think you can let it slide. It must still be considered an emergency, even if you consider it minor, or if you've gotten used to it. Pain is the body's chief, although often delayed, warning device, and you should always heed that warning.

- ☐ **Swelling or lump** Any swelling, lump, or tenderness in the jaw or gum region usually indicates either an abscessed tooth (especially if it's in the area of the jaw where the roots of the teeth are located) or an abscess of the gum pocket. It could also indicate a more serious condition, like a tumor. The area may be tender, but not necessarily painful. So, even if there's no pain, the condition must be dealt with immediately.

- ☐ **Bleeding** Bleeding around the teeth or gums, whether it's constant or occasional, usually indicates gum disease, although you can have severe periodontitis and not see any bleeding (until you have hygiene therapy). But bleeding isn't limited to gum disease. It could very well be an indicator of another, more serious disease. If you have bleeding, even if you think you know the cause of it, you should be examined, diagnosed, and treated immediately.

- ☐ **Odor** A strong, fetid, putrid odor is another symptom of an emergency, though not often thought of as such. In most cases this odor is symptomatic of acute gum disease. I'm not talking about garlic or cigarette breath, which disappears when the cause is eliminated.

TYPES OF DENTAL EMERGENCIES
AND WHAT TO DO ABOUT THEM

Although you need to have any dental emergency checked out by a dentist, the following suggestions can often help relieve the pain and discomfort of the most common types of emergencies. *Remember, relieving a symptom is not a cure and will not remove the cause of the problem.*

Decay

Decay is the number one cause of dental emergencies. It can happen to any tooth, but the bottom line is the same: pain, ranging from a dull, throbbing ache to out-and-out acute (sudden and intense) pain. Usually you'll recognize a tooth decay emergency because the tooth in question will be sensitive to pressure, heat or cold, or food and drink that are acidic or that contain sugar. Toothache from decay can come and go, so don't think you're out of the woods if the pain goes away on its own. A one-time trauma to a tooth, such as might be caused by biting down on something hard, may get your attention, but this type of pain will soon subside (unless you break or fracture the tooth or filling). The trick here is to know that if there's no obvious reason for the pain, you most likely have decay, and the pain is trying to tell you to do something about it.

Home treatment There are various ways of treating a decay emergency at home. Here are a few of the more effective methods.

OIL OF CLOVES The very best home remedy is Orajel. It contains oil of cloves, a great nerve sedative, and an anesthetic to relieve pain. You can get it at just about any drugstore. It's a good idea to keep it on hand, since the drugstore isn't always open when a decay emergency occurs. But I recommend it only as a temporary measure because even if it reduces or removes the symptoms it will not *cure* decay.

The first thing to do is determine if there's any opening you can see. Use your penlight-mirror (see pages 58–59) and check it out. If there's any food stuck in the opening, try to remove it. A toothpick is the best instrument. Avoid using any object that is metallic, like a safety pin, because the dentin and exposed nerves are extremely sensitive to metal. Never poke too hard—if the cavity is deep and close to the pulp you can perforate the pulp. Lightly move the toothpick around the cavity, and if the food doesn't come out easily, leave it be.

Next, saturate a small piece of absorbent cotton or cloth with Orajel or oil of cloves and gently place it in the opening if there is one, or dab the cotton in the most susceptible areas (on the top of the tooth, at the contact point, or around the gum line). Tweezers may work well, if you have the dexterity and the access. If there's an opening but it's too small to put anything into it, you may be able to squeeze a few drops of the oil from the cloth into the hole. Then cover the area with a piece of untreated cotton, gauze, or cloth, and hold it in place with your finger, or place light pressure with the opposite tooth. Don't use your tongue as the holder because the oil may irritate it.

Even if you don't have oil of cloves, it's essential to cover the exposed area in order to keep out air and food, especially irritating liquids.

TEMPORARY FILLING MATERIAL There's a temporary filling material that you can purchase at the drugstore called DenTemp. It's a good idea to have this product in your medicine cabinet because a toothache can occur at any time. Follow the directions on the label, dry the cavity with a piece of cotton or tissue, and insert the DenTemp into the opening—by itself or over the cotton soaked in oil of cloves. This will help seal off the exposed area and prevent food and air from entering the cavity. Again, this is only a temporary emergency treatment, and even if it relieves the symptoms, you should see a dentist as soon as possible. A word of caution: it's possible that the tooth could be abscessed. When you seal it, you may feel pressure building or an intensification of pain. If this happens, remove the temporary filling.

ASPIRIN Take a pain pill. Aspirin seems to be most effective for toothaches (I recommend Bufferin), but take whatever you prefer. *Do not ever*, and I repeat, *ever*, place an aspirin in your mouth without swallowing it. Aspirin is very acidic and is strong enough to actually burn the gums and other soft tissues of your mouth. Besides, aspirin won't give any pain relief when placed on the tooth. In fact, if it contacts the exposed part of the dentin or nerve, it could cause you more pain than the decay. Your good intentions will just compound the problem.

A *few cautions* If you must eat before your aching tooth is treated, don't eat anything that is hard or sticky, too hot or too cold. Definitely avoid chewing on the side that is affected. The best thing is to take only liquids and to use a straw.

Definitely don't eat anything with sugar in it—it'll be like stepping on the tooth's nerve. Don't forget, sugar is what probably caused the problem in the first place.

Be careful not to breathe through your mouth because the nerve is extremely sensitive to air, particularly cold air, and it'll only aggravate the situation.

Wisdom Teeth

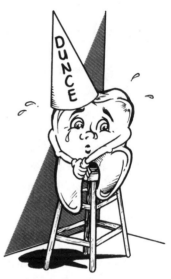

Wisdom teeth aren't really so smart. If they were, they wouldn't be the number two cause of dental emergencies. (See illustration on page 35.) Most wisdom teeth end up being extracted. The reason for this is they rarely come in properly. And there are two main reasons for *that*. One: because we no longer eat the type of diet our ancestors ate, over time our jaws have become smaller, but we still have the same number of teeth trying to fit into a smaller space. Genetics is the other reason. The offspring of a large person and a small person will often end up with a small jaw and large teeth. Because of the lack of jaw space, wisdom teeth often only partially erupt, are impacted into the jawbone, or come in tilted. If they don't erupt normally they won't mesh with their opposing partner, and if they don't meet properly they'll be ineffective for chewing. If they can't chew for you, they're about as valuable as a car with no tires. Wisdom teeth are also the most difficult teeth to keep clean, are not naturally self-cleansing, and are the hardest to see. All of which means they're an accident waiting to happen and are prime candidates for an emergency.

The immediate cause of this emergency is usually decay, gum infection, or *pericoronitis* (an infection generally caused by food and plaque getting stuck under the flap of skin that covers a portion of the chewing surface of a partially erupted wisdom tooth).

Your dentist can tell you if you're one of the very few who have normal, healthy, and functional wisdom teeth. If that's the case, you can certainly keep them . . . but remember, they'll still need a lot of care. If your wisdom teeth haven't erupted properly, the best way to deal with them is to have them pulled before the emergency takes place. If you have them removed when there is no infection, and you're in good health, the extraction procedure and recovery will most likely be fine. On the other hand, once they become badly decayed, or the gums become infected, the extraction process not only becomes more difficult for you, but the odds of an uneventful recovery decrease dramatically.

Home treatment If you have decay symptoms in your wisdom teeth, follow the instructions for dealing with decay in the last section. If the gums are red, swollen, and tender to the touch, here's what you can do at home. Mix a 3 percent solution of hydrogen peroxide with an equal amount of warm water. Take a mouthful of the mixture and bathe the affected area by gently swishing it over the tender spot. Do this for two to three minutes. Spit it out, wait about fifteen minutes and then rinse with warm saltwater (one-half teaspoon of salt in about four ounces of warm water) for two to three minutes. Follow this procedure two or three times, and then wait a half hour to see if it brings you any relief.

You can also take some aspirin if you're in a lot of discomfort. But remember—these procedures are only meant to give you some relief until you can get to the dentist. The pain will keep returning until you get the problem treated.

Emergency Extractions

If you go to the dentist for an emergency and a decision is made to extract a tooth, he may decide to put you on antibiotics prior to the extraction. Normally antibiotics aren't used unless there's infection in the gums around the tooth or an abscess in the bone surrounding the tip of the root. If you're not protected by antibiotic therapy, the infection could spread to your bloodstream. Since your resistance has already been lowered because of the infection, it's not worth taking that risk. So if there's infection, I suggest you don't have the tooth extracted unless you're protected by antibiotics or the infection has subsided. Always take the full course of antibiotics prescribed, even if your tooth feels fine after a few days, or you run the risk of the bacteria becoming resistant to the antibiotic. Not good.

Once the tooth has been extracted, the dentist will give you written instructions for home care. Don't leave the office without *written* instructions, and follow them to the letter, no matter how easily the procedure went or how good you may feel afterward.

Broken Teeth

If a tooth is partially or completely broken off, pain (exposed nerves) and bleeding are usually the first things you'll want to deal with. Even if the tooth is just fractured, you could still have pain, and the self-treatment is the same. Take a small piece of the cleanest material you have available to you—absorbent cotton, gauze, or even a piece of shirt or other material. Soak it in your mouth until it's warm and moistened. Or, if you can, run it under warm water. Place it over the broken tooth and bite down gently to hold it in place. Besides stanching the flow of blood, this will serve to help immobilize the tooth if it's loose. Don't bite down any harder than is necessary because you don't want to be putting excessive pressure on it. Keep your mouth closed as much as possible and talk as little as you have to. Take whatever pain relievers you normally take, if needed.

Get in touch with your dentist. If you can't reach him, ask his answering service to put you in touch with whoever is handling his emergency calls, or go to the yellow pages and get an emergency appointment with another dentist.

Burns

Burns of the mouth are very common, and some can be serious enough to require immediate treatment. Generally, after the cause of the burn is removed or the affected area flushed with water (if the burn is caused by a chemical such as aspirin or Clorox), the wound will heal by itself, although it may be tender for a while.

Hot food, hot liquids, or chemicals Often you'll be more aware of burns from heat or chemicals the day after the burn than at the time it occurred. The pain is often delayed until the burned skin sloughs off, usually the next day, exposing the tender, sensitive skin underneath. Rinsing the area with body-temperature water usually helps relieve the tenderness. But if it's not too painful it'll heal faster if it's bathed in saliva. Orajel also makes a product to help relieve burn symptoms. It's called Mouth-Aid.

The pain may be minimal until the exposed skin comes in contact with something you put in your mouth. Also, you can irritate it when you swallow or speak. When you discover a movement that irritates the wound, avoid that movement as much as possible. Swallowing, of course, is an exception. Try to keep your tongue away from the burn. You can help your situation out by not subjecting the wounded area to hot, irritating, or acid food and drink. If you smoke it would be a good idea to stop until it heals.

Check out the burn with your mouth mirror to follow its progress. If it's uncomfortable but doesn't need medical attention it should heal in seven to ten days, but if it doesn't, you should consult your dentist or doctor. There are numerous medications he can prescribe for you.

Aspirin burns Aspirin (especially if it's crushed) placed directly against the gums, if you leave it there long enough, can burn the gums and other soft tissues of the mouth. The best treatment is to rinse with warm water. Once you stop the aspirin input, the affected tissue will normally heal itself.

Cuts

Many minor cuts of the lip, cheek, or tongue can be treated at home. Whatever the cause, the first concern is to clean the wound and stop the bleeding. If the cut is on the lip, rinse it well with water, dry it, and put a bandaid, or tape, over it to close the wound. If you can place ice over the cut, prior to placing the bandaid, it'll help stop the bleeding, reduce swelling, and relieve the pain. Leave the ice on for fifteen minutes, then remove it for fifteen minutes. Doing this for thirty to sixty minutes should keep the swelling down.

If the cut is on the cheek or tongue, the best way to stop the bleeding is with pressure. You can do this with your finger, a piece of gauze, or a tea bag soaked in water. Tea contains tannic acid, which helps constrict blood vessels.

As with any cut, on any part of your body, you must be concerned about infection. At the first sign of infection (increased redness, swelling, pain, or pus), you should contact your dentist.

Jaw or Facial Fractures

If you receive a blow to the jaw or face and think you may have fractured something, there are two things you must do. First, *immediately* call an oral surgeon or go to the emergency ward of the closest hospital. Second, keep your jaw or face immobilized. Find the most comfortable position you can and don't move the affected part. You don't have to open your jaw to talk; speak through your teeth.

IN SUMMARY

This chapter gives you the basic information you need to determine whether you have an emergency and what to do about it. But even if you're not sure it's an emergency you should act as if it is. "But why?" you say. "What if I go running to the dentist and it's not an emergency after all?" Well, when it comes to dental emergencies, it's better to be safe than sorry. And what's the worst thing that could happen? Your dentist tells you to relax, it's nothing that serious. That in itself should make your trip to the dentist well worth it.

When you call the dental office, be sure and tell whomever you speak to that you truly believe you have an emergency. Most receptionists and dentists try to screen such calls. They'll try to determine if you really do have one, or if you have a problem that can wait for a regularly scheduled visit. That's a good policy because it could save you an unnecessary trip. But if, after their screening, you still feel you have a real emergency, be adamant about coming in.

Please note that none of the home remedies I've suggested are meant as a permanent treatment or repair. May you live long and prosper and never have an emergency.

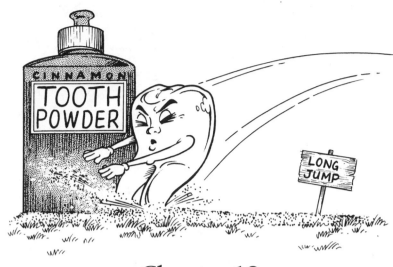

Chapter 12

Dental Specialists

It was a big step for humankind when barber-dentists dropped their combs and razors and became dentists only. For one thing, it meant there would no longer be hair on the floor when they worked on someone's teeth. It was just as big a step when dentists began to specialize. It was also a logical step, and one that has positively benefited the dental patient.

Today, like it or not, we live in the age of specialization. For the most part specialization has been advantageous to the patient, and to the dental profession as well. It has directly led to the development of new equipment, new techniques, and new materials. What this means to you is better treatment.

Every general dentist has some training in each of the specialized areas of dental treatment, and in many cases your dentist can provide you with the same quality treatment as the specialist. But there's a point at which he won't be able to offer you the same skill and experience. Most dentists are aware of what they can and cannot do and will refer you to a specialist when necessary . . . but it never hurts to ask. Whenever your dentist wants to work in any of the specialized areas, there's only one question I'd want you to ask him: "Doc, if this was your mouth and you needed this procedure done, would you refer yourself to the specialist?"

HOW TO FIND A SPECIALIST

In most cases a specialist will be recommended to you by your general dentist. This is the best place to start because your dentist will have established a good working relationship with a specialist from each field. If you don't have a regular dentist and feel you need to see a specialist, you can follow the same procedures I talked about in Chapter 6 ("Finding a Dentist and a Dental Hygienist"). But it's always a good idea to consult with a general dentist before seeing a specialist, unless it's for emergency treatment.

THE ORTHODONTIST

The orthodontist is trained in the highly specialized branch of dentistry called *orthodontics*. Orthodontics deals with straightening out teeth that are not in proper alignment (are rotated, tilted, etc.), correcting bite problems, and aligning jaws. For the most part, this treatment is done to restore your mouth to normal health and function, but it can also be done for purely cosmetic, or aesthetic, reasons. I feel that orthodontics is one of the most positive aspects of modern dentistry. Having properly aligned teeth that close together in the right way is very important both to your general health, because it enables you to efficiently chew your food, and to the health of your mouth specifically because it makes your oral hygiene much easier.

When to See an Orthodontist

Anybody, at any age, may be a candidate for orthodontic treatment. But when orthodontic problems are caught early, they are easier to treat, take less time, and are much less expensive. If you're a parent this means you should have your kids' teeth checked out as soon as possible.

Adults Orthodontics for adults is no more difficult to do than for children, given the same situation, and no matter what you've believed in the past, you're never too old for it. However, as with children, the sooner you start treatment the easier it will be on your teeth and on your wallet.

Children If the orthodontist has a chance to examine the child at an early age, about the time the lower front (baby) teeth come in, he can often predict (by taking measurements of both jaw and tooth sizes and projecting their growth rate) if your child will have orthodontic problems when all the permanent teeth have arrived. If he feels there'll be problems, he can perform what's called *preventive* or *interceptive orthodontics*. Often this means that he'll be able to reduce the extent of the brace work or totally eliminate the need for braces later on. It's also possible that the orthodontist may only need to perform "selective serial extractions," the removal of one or more teeth, to allow enough space for the permanent teeth to come in. In some cases, this is all that's needed to correct a problem that—untreated—could cost you many thousands of dollars, and your child a great deal of trauma, later on. Some background information should help you get a better understanding about the value of orthodontic treatment.

Bite Problems

Facial contours, the size of the jaw, and tooth size are all hereditary (or, in rare cases, disease-related). The orthodontist may talk to you about the relationship between jaw and tooth size. For example, if a child inherits her mom's small jaw and her father's large teeth, the end result may be teeth that are too big for her jaw.

This overcrowding is a serious problem. It can prevent some teeth from erupting and cause the crowding or partial impaction of others. (An *impacted* tooth is one that does not erupt normally but is completely or partially buried in the jawbone or partially covered by gum tissue.) It also results in an abnormal bite, called *malocclusion* by the dental profession. Teeth should be like well-adjusted gears; they should join in harmony to distribute the forces of chewing evenly over all of the teeth. When they're overcrowded and misaligned, they're like gears that have jammed up and don't function well, if at all. Malocclusion can result in many problems:

- ☐ Excessive trauma to and stress on the teeth, ligaments, jaw joints and muscles, and the jawbone
- ☐ Speech difficulties
- ☐ Hard-to-clean teeth
- ☐ Inefficient chewing and digestion

☐ Acceleration of gum disease, bone loss, TMJ problems, and ultimately the premature loss of teeth

Is It Worth the Cost?

It is always better to fix the fence before the horse takes off. It's cheaper too, because you won't end up losing the horse.

Every situation in orthodontics is different, so don't compare your situation to someone else's. If you're a parent, don't worry about what another parent may tell you. Rather, find out from an orthodontist where your child stands in the scheme of orthodontic treatment. You can help by keeping an eye on your child's oral development. Check her mouth against the charts and drawings on pages 272–73 in Chapter 17, "Parent and Child." The key here is *prevention*: the earlier you get your child (or yourself) checked out, the easier and less costly the work will be. If you think that there's no point in looking into it because you simply can't afford extensive orthodontic treatment, it may still be worth the small price of the exam. You may discover that the treatment won't be as expensive as you imagined it would be. And your orthodontist may provide a payment plan that fits into your budget.

Turning out smiles that look like a set of ivories is not the main purpose of orthodontics. There's much more to it than that. Every dollar spent in correcting the problem at an early age will prevent worse problems later on . . . and *save* you lots of money. Not to mention your teeth.

THE ORAL SURGEON

If you're like most people, you probably think that all an oral surgeon does is remove teeth. That he does; but extracting teeth is only one of many valuable services he provides. Of all the dental specialists, the oral surgeon undergoes the most extensive training. Because his areas of expertise are not limited to treating the teeth and gums, I see him as the bridge between the medical and dental branches of medicine. The oral surgeon does the following:

☐ Treats jaw and facial fractures

☐ Performs reconstructive surgery for the repair of damage to the oral cavity due to injuries, cancer, and genetic defects such as cleft palates

☐ Diagnoses and treats oral cancers and cysts of the mouth, jaws, and face

☐ Assists the orthodontist with the surgical procedures required to reposition the jaws to correct severe malocclusions

☐ Works closely with the general dentist and prosthodontist (see pages 224–25) in making certain types of dentures

☐ Performs implant surgery

☐ Works in the field of pain management, including injuries to the nerves of the teeth, mouth, and face

☐ Diagnoses and treats TMJ problems

☐ Diagnoses and treats injuries and diseases of the tongue and salivary glands

☐ Administers general anesthesia

I hope you never need him, but isn't it nice to know he's there?

Because of his extensive training he is best suited to handle any difficult oral-facial surgery, but he's not the only dental professional who is trained and qualified to extract teeth. The general dentist can provide this service. What isn't always so easy for you to figure out is when to use the oral surgeon and when to use your dentist. Although most dentists feel comfortable with routine extractions, my suggestion is to have wisdom teeth and other complicated extractions done by the oral surgeon. The general rule of thumb is to ask your dentist if he considers the extraction complicated and would he have the oral surgeon extract the tooth if it were his own.

THE ENDODONTIST (Root Canal Specialist)

Endodontists specialize in treating problems of the tooth's nerves and blood vessels, both of which are located in the pulp and root canal (see illustration on page 46). Advanced decay and trauma to the tooth's nerves are the most common cause of that infamous procedure known as a *root canal*, which I'll explain in a moment. When the decay reaches the tooth's dentin, the dentin is exposed to germs and their toxins. If caught soon enough, via dental exam or X ray, the decay can be removed and the tooth filled without further damage. But if the decay is allowed to proceed it will eventually reach the pulp and destroy it. Then the infection will proceed into the root canal. Because the root canal is so narrow, any infection causing inflammation and swelling will give you intense pain. But you must remember that pain will not *always* be present; it may not show up until the bone around the root tip has also become infected, and sometimes not even then.

Whether or not there's pain, once the pulp has been infected and is dying, either a root canal must be done or the tooth will have to be removed. In a root canal, in order to remove the infection, the contents of the pulp and root canal are completely removed. If this isn't done, the germs, and the resulting infection, can travel down the root canal and infect the bone that surrounds the root. This not only destroys the bone but can cause an abscess, intense pain, and swelling in the area around the root. This isn't a happy occurrence; it can be one of the most painful dental experiences you may ever experience.

The endodontist is specially trained to treat such infections and traumas to the pulp and root canal. He removes the infection and fills the canal or canals (teeth may have one, two, or three roots) with a special material. Sometimes the infection is so bad that the endodontist must drill through the jawbone in order to remove the infection around the root tip. Sometimes part of the root tip itself will have to be removed. This is called *apico-surgery*, or an *apicoectomy*.

The most important thing I can tell you about the endodontist is that he can help you save an infected tooth from extraction. And if you can save an infected tooth you can also save the cost of the bridge that would have been needed to replace that tooth. If you think that a root canal is expensive, remember that it'll never be as expensive as replacing the tooth. A three-unit bridge needed to replace one tooth could be two to three times as expensive as a root canal.

After the root canal is done, it's back to your general dentist. Now, depending on how much of the tooth is left, several things can be done to restore the tooth. You may only need a little filling. Or the tooth may need a full crown, if the destruction has been severe. Sometimes the tooth may be so decayed that, after the root canal is done, there's not enough tooth structure left to support a crown. In this case the dentist has to place a post into the root and build up a filling around it in order to support a crown.

Any time a root canal has been done, and the tooth's pulp and root canal have been cleaned out, the tooth is more susceptible to fracturing because the tooth dries out when the nerves and blood vessels no longer provide it with fluids. So, if your dentist tells you a tooth with a root canal needs to be crowned to keep it from fracturing, you now know why.

THE PERIODONTIST

The periodontist is the dentist who treats periodontal disease after it has gone beyond what you and the dental hygienist can treat with in-office hygiene therapy and home care. He may be the only one who can help you save your teeth if you have reached that stage. (If he can't, the next stop is the oral surgeon's office.) The periodontist is highly qualified to perform the various types of periodontal surgery that may be necessary to remove infected gum tissue, to remove infection from the bone, and to recontour the bone so that you can more easily keep the now more vulnerable gums and teeth clean.

Both your dental hygienist and dentist will monitor your gum disease to determine whether you can keep your teeth and gums clean enough to prevent the disease from advancing without periodontal surgery. Often, once you're practicing proper hygiene, you'll find that some areas won't need surgery at all, and others will need less than first expected. But if you do need periodontal surgery, there are two very important things you should know:

- ☐ You shouldn't have the surgery done until you have first been given the opportunity to see what you and your hygienist can do to treat the problem. (Emergency surgery is an exception.) Having your gums as healthy as you can get them before surgery will greatly speed up the after-surgery healing.

- ☐ Any periodontal surgery that removes gum tissue and bone also creates food traps that never existed before. Since whatever you did to take care of your teeth before you got gum disease didn't work (or you wouldn't have gotten it), logic says that the same appraoch to oral hygiene definitely won't work when you no longer have the natural protection the bone and gums once provided. If you're going to have periodontal surgery done—and I can't stress this enough—you must be willing to establish not only a new attitude toward your oral health but a new oral hygiene program as well. Surgery may take care of the immediate problem, but you'll soon be back where you started—unless you are willing to devote whatever time and energy it takes to keep your gums free of disease.

Your periodontist will give you instructions on home care, and you must follow them to the letter. Both the periodontist and the hygienist will provide you with, or will have you purchase, special preventive aids, such as perio-brushes, perio-picks, and even prescription mouthwashes. Make sure you use them religiously. If you don't, you can say good-bye to your teeth.

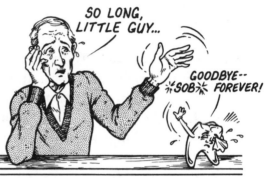

THE PROSTHODONTIST

Not many people know what a prosthodontist does, if they've heard of him at all. The prosthodontist is a specialist in making crowns, bridges, and dentures. In the trade, he is also called a "crown and bridge specialist" or a "denture specialist," depending on which particular sort of dental hardware he specializes in making. While general dentists can handle most tooth replacements, prosthodontists are trained to deal with the more challenging problems. They're experienced in handling complicated TMJ and bite problems and often work hand in hand with the orthodontist and the oral surgeon on difficult cases. They also deal with:

- ☐ Severe bruxism and night grinding problems
- ☐ Severe injury or cancer patients who need extensive dental reconstruction
- ☐ Severe periodontal cases where specialized crown and bridge or partial denture work is needed to stabilize teeth that can no longer hold up on their own.

□ Severe cosmetic cases where extensive anterior bridge work is needed not only to restore the front teeth to function but to make them cosmetically pleasing as well

□ Implants

DR. TOM'S TIPS

Specialists are a valuable addition to dentistry. Any good dentist, if he feels a case is too difficult for him, will refer you to the one you'll need. In this, he is like your oral health coordinator, making sure you will get the best treatment possible by directing you to the appropriate specialist. Heed his advice, but always make sure you're clear about why he is referring you and what you can expect when you get there.

THE PEDIATRIC DENTIST

Everything you need to know about pediatric dentistry can be found on pages 282–85, in Chapter 17, "Parent and Child."

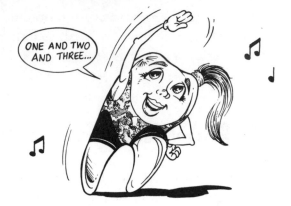

ONE AND TWO AND THREE...

Chapter 13

Looking Good: Cosmetic Dentistry

Cosmetic dentistry is pretty much what the name implies, dentistry that makes you look better. More accurately, cosmetic dentistry makes your teeth look better. And if your teeth look better you feel better.

Cosmetic dentistry, also referred to as *aesthetic dentistry*, has always been a part of the practice of dentistry, even though the choices available to you in the past were expensive and limited. Recently there have been tremendous advances in materials and techniques, and cosmetic dentistry has now become one of most innovative and exciting fields of modern dentistry.

WHAT IT IS

Cosmetic dentistry can be used to correct a variety of problems—some of which could have been prevented, and others that could not. For example:

1. Stains caused by food and drink

2. Stains caused by drugs or chemicals

3. Yellowed teeth

4. Pits and defects

5. Genetic abnormalities like overlapped teeth and gaps between the teeth

6. Worn or chipped teeth

7. Unsightly amalgam fillings

Many new or improved materials are used in cosmetic dentistry today that weren't available in the past, and new ones appear all the time. They range from high-tech composite resins, porcelain veneers, and specialized resin bonding (adhesive) materials all the way to twenty-first-century bleaching agents, to name a few.

Compared to today's methods the traditional approach, crowning teeth (which is discussed in Chapter 14, "Restorations"), was more costly, required the removal of more tooth structure, and took more in-office time. It also sometimes caused irreversible damage to the tooth's pulp. Today, in most cases, the fantastic new materials available mean that you can restore both function and aesthetics but in a less expensive and time-consuming way, with less damage to the tooth.

When you sit down with your dentist to discuss treatment plans you should tell him you want not only to have the necessary repair done but also, whenever financially possible, to restore or improve your original appearance. Ask your dentist to evaluate whether cosmetic dentistry makes sense in your particular case. Have him explain the trade-offs in terms of cost and durability, as compared to the more traditional porcelain or acrylic crowns.

I can't tell you what type of cosmetic dentistry might be best for you—that will be between you and the doc—but when you finish this chapter you'll know if it's something you want to consider and what your choices and alternatives are. With that in mind, let's take a look at what you should know in order to make an educated decision.

FINDING THE RIGHT COSMETIC DENTIST

The best way to find a good cosmetic dentist is to ask a friend who has found a good one. Ask him how he likes what's been done and check out the results yourself. You can also write or call the American Academy of Cosmetic Dentistry (2709 Marshall, Madison, Wisconsin 53705, 608-238-2300) and ask if there's a member dentist practicing in your area. Another way to find one is to look in the yellow pages. You'll see that some dentists advertise the fact that they do cosmetic restorations and others don't. This is a place to start, but use it as a guide, not the gospel. Cosmetic dentistry isn't a recognized dental specialty, so if you do use the yellow pages, remember that if a dentist advertises that he does cosmetic dentistry it doesn't necessarily mean he does a lot of it or is good at it. Whichever approach you use, follow the guidelines outlined in Chapter 6, "Finding a Dentist and a Dental Hygienist."

The fact that it takes skill and practice to master the techniques of cosmetic dentistry means that it's important to select a dentist who keeps up-to-date on the latest materials, techniques, and equipment. Ask your dentist how much of his practice is devoted to cosmetic dentistry. If he tells you it's only a small percentage, ask him to give you the name of a dentist who does a lot of it. If he tells you he likes doing it, attends workshops and seminars, and performs a lot of cosmetic treatment, ask him to show you before and after photographs of work he has done. Don't settle for before and after shots of another dentist's work or promotional photographs from a cosmetic product manufacturer.

BONDING (Veneering)

To restore the beauty and function of teeth, cosmetic dentists use a method they call *bonding*, or *veneering*. This technique is used to cover up defects, severe stains, chips, or fractures. It's also used to build up a tooth that's too small, to fill in space between teeth that are too far apart, or to recontour a tooth.

Depending on the extent of the bonding and how well you take care of your mouth, the repair can last five years, or even longer. However, because every situation varies, no dentist can accurately predict its longevity, even though techniques and materials have improved vastly over the last few years. The really nice thing about bonding is that, in most cases, if a piece breaks off, the tooth can be easily touched up.

Three types of veneers are used: porcelain, acrylic (plastic), and composite. All of them are bonded (attached) to the tooth with a cementlike material.

Porcelain and Acrylic (Plastic) Veneers

The porcelain veneer is a very thin shell of porcelain, custom-made from an impression of the tooth (or teeth) it will be placed on. It's also known as a "custom veneer." Usually two visits to the dentist are required to put a porcelain veneer in place. First, some of the tooth may have to be removed or reshaped, but even in these instances much less tooth structure is lost for a veneer than for a crown. Then an impression of the tooth is taken. Next, the veneer itself is made at the lab.

When it's done, the dentist cements it onto the tooth at a subsequent visit. The first step in this process is to etch, or roughen, the tooth's surface so that the bonding material will adhere better. Then a liquid bonding material is applied to the tooth's surface, and the veneer is put in place. Finally the edges are shaped, smoothed, and polished, and—presto!—you have what looks like a new tooth.

Unlike their porcelain counterparts, acrylic veneers are pre-made and known as "prefabricated veneers." Both types are bonded to the tooth in basically the same way.

Composite Veneers

Composite veneers, usually simply called composites, are bonded to the tooth in a totally different way than the porcelain or acrylic veneers. Whereas the other veneers are like false fingernails placed on top of the real ones, the composite veneer is like fingernail polish that is painted on the nail.

The same initial etching process takes place, but after the tooth has been roughened, the pastelike composite resin is applied directly to the tooth. Then it's contoured to the shape of the tooth. Once it's close to the desired form, it is hardened either by a chemical reaction or with the use of a special fiber-optic light. Then the finishing shaping touches are made, and finally it's smoothed and polished to a natural, toothlike luster. Usually this is a one-visit procedure.

Composites can also be used as a filling material for repairing decay in teeth. Until recently it was only used for small fillings, but due to advances in composite materials some products now claim to be hard and durable enough to be used for larger fillings, including fillings involving chewing surfaces.

A Comparison

Porcelain veneers offer some distinct advantages over both acrylic and composite restorations.

- ☐ They look more lifelike. The color match is better, and so is color stability. They're shinier and smoother, and the translucency of porcelain makes it look more natural.
- ☐ They won't stain.
- ☐ They last longer.
- ☐ They resist abrasion better than acrylic.

On the other hand, acrylic and composite veneers are usually less expensive and resist edge fracturing better than porcelain veneers. The choice of the bonding material will be determined by the condition of the individual tooth. Your dentist will give you your options based on cost, aesthetics, and durability.

Bonding is not the only way to improve a tooth's appearance. In many cases a tooth can be whitened by bleaching.

BLEACHING

The bleaching of teeth has been going on for over one hundred years. When done right it can be a safe, inexpensive, and aesthetic way to whiten teeth. In the last few years the techniques and bleaching materials have improved dramatically, and I predict the trend will continue.

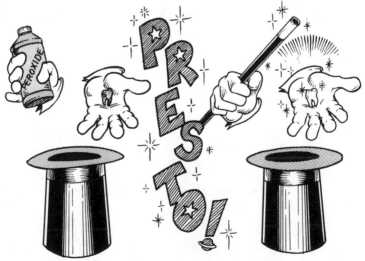

The most effective active ingredient for bleaching teeth has long been hydrogen peroxide (H_2O_2). It's available in many different concentrations (percent of hydrogen peroxide in the bleaching solution) and can be applied in different ways. Although it's most effective at bleaching superficial stains of the enamel, it also has the ability, when applied correctly and over a long enough period of time, to penetrate through the enamel and dissolve deeper stains found within the dentin.

Although no one, including the dentist, can guarantee how successful bleaching will be, costwise it should always be considered as the first alternative. If bleaching doesn't give you the results you seek, you can always move on to the next level of cosmetically treating your teeth, such as bonding or porcelain crowns. But when compared to crowns, for example, not only is bleaching the less expensive way to go but less tooth structure is lost.

There are two approaches to bleaching your teeth. The first is at the dental office, and the second is at home.

At the Dental Office

In my opinion, the best and most efficient way to bleach your teeth is at the dental office. Dentists who specialize in this are up-to-date and knowledgeable about the kinds of bleaching agents available. Because they have better ways to control the application and protect the gums and other soft tissues of the mouth from the bleaching agent's potentially harmful effects, they can use much stronger concentrations of hydrogen peroxide than are legally available to the do-it-yourselfer. Bleaching done at the dental office is also faster, produces a more even effect, and usually will last longer than bleaching done at home. The amount of time it will take to produce the desired lightening will depend on how deeply the tooth is stained and, if office bleaching is supported by home application, how diligently you follow the instructions. When done in conjunction with home bleaching, where the bleaching agent is left on six to eight hours a day (depending on the method used), results can be seen in a few days, with the most noticeable difference seen in two to three weeks.

The dentist has a great deal of experience in determining which teeth are good candidates for bleaching and which will get better results with bonded veneers or composites. The dentist will also know the most effective bleaching agent and method of application to use for your unique situation.

Home Bleaching

If you watch TV you already know that tooth-whitening products are a hot item, especially for the newest form of TV advertising, called infomercials. Some products require a *mouth-guard* (a flexible device designed to keep the bleach in contact with the tooth, and from leaking onto the gum tissue), and others don't use one. Some brands claim you only need to apply the bleaching agent for a few minutes per day, while others suggest that their product may need to be used for up to three hundred hours. The amount of hydrogen peroxide that is released varies with each brand, and the results you get will depend on:

- ☐ The amount of time the bleaching agent is in contact with the tooth
- ☐ The concentration of peroxide in the bleaching agent
- ☐ How long you use the product
- ☐ The type and severity of the stain
- ☐ The location of the stain

If you're going to do it on your own, you should be aware that home bleaching, unless you first get an evaluation by the dentist, is not nearly as predictable as office bleaching. One reason over-the-counter bleaches fail to get good results is that unless you can accurately diagnosis the original cause of the stain, you can't determine the best method of treatment for removing it. The stain could be caused by decay, amalgam fillings, or even a tooth that is dying, and in these cases bleaching may not be the treatment of choice. If you don't check with your dentist first you may be wasting your time and money using bleaching agents to remove stains on teeth that should be treated with veneers, composites, or crowns.

I'm not saying that the over-the-counter approach will never work (in some cases they work very well)—only that you'd be better off if you first got your dentist's opinion. Even if you don't want him to do the bleaching, you should ask him if the tooth (or teeth) is a candidate for bleaching and to recommend the best over-the-counter product for your situation. Dentists have access to all the latest research and materials and will give you more objective information than any advertisement. If you don't have a dentist, want to go it alone, and are willing to accept the consequences of your decision (that your efforts may be in vain), I recommend the Rembrandt Lightening Gel system.

No matter what brand you choose, follow the directions explicitly. Irresponsible use of the solution, depending on what system is used, could cause excessive etching of the enamel, irritation of the soft tissues, tooth sensitivity, uneven whitening, and, if swallowed, sore throat, diarrhea, and nausea. Never use any whitening system if you're allergic to any of its ingredients, especially hydrogen peroxide and glycerin. Even though it may not say so on the package, I don't believe any bleach should be used during pregnancy or while breast-feeding because studies to determine its safety have not been done.

Bleaching Toothpastes

I've already spoken in detail about toothpastes (see Chapter 4). In general they're the least effective method of bleaching your teeth, but when used in conjunction with a professional bleaching procedure, a whitening toothpaste may help the bleaching last longer. Rembrandt toothpaste, in my opinion, is the best of this type of toothpaste, especially when used with Rembrandt Lightening Gel. (However, remember that my recommendations are not a diagnosis. If your dentist recommends another product, take his advice. If what he recommends is different than mine and doesn't work, then you can give my suggestions a try.)

TIPS AND TIDBITS

1. Serious tooth grinders and clenchers are often not the best candidates for bonded veneers. These habits place great stress on the restoration and can lead to fractures. If you're a grinder or clencher be sure to mention this to your dentist. Perhaps bleaching will be the method of choice for you.

2. Bleaching can be done on any tooth and at any age.

3. When done correctly bleaching is a very safe procedure; there have been no reports of permanent damage to the tooth's

nerve. However, sometimes it can cause nerve sensitivity. Many dentists will do a topical fluoride treatment or use other methods to alleviate the sensitivity. The important thing is to tell your dentist if you're experiencing sensitivity so he can do something about it.

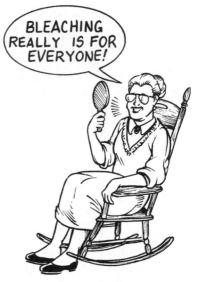

4. It's impossible to predict the results of bleaching, and not everyone will get the results they seek. This is especially true if the results you're hoping for aren't realistic or if you're not willing to make the effort that long-term bleaching requires. Also, if you have overly sensitive teeth or extremely dark and deep stains, you may not get the degree of whitening you desire. You may end up needing to have bonded veneers done in order to achieve your goal.

5. Remember—bleaching isn't usually permanent. The discoloration can return over time, and rebleaching will often be necessary. If a tooth is discolored because it has died, you may need to repeat the bleaching procedure every two to three years.

6. Some bleaching procedures involve using a mouth-guard while you sleep. If you also wear it during the day, you can speed up the bleaching process.

7. Irritation to the gums will be proportional to the concentration of hydrogen peroxide and acids in the bleaching solution and the amount of time the solution is in contact with the gums and other soft tissues of the mouth. The chance of irritation is eliminated, or drastically reduced, if the mouth-guard is custom-made at the dental office.

8. Bleaching is safe for restorations because it doesn't negatively affect any of the filling materials.

9. The hydrogen peroxide used in some at-home bleaching treatments has the side benefit of reducing the mouth's bacterial count.

10. *Acid etching* is a method using acid to etch off superficial stains that have not deeply penetrated the enamel. Once the tooth is etched, it's smoothed and polished. This technique works well for some fluoride stains, because most of these are in the outer portion of the enamel or in small, isolated areas.

11. Because of children's tendency to swallow much of what they put in their mouth, I suggest you don't attempt home bleaching on your child's teeth unless your dentist okays it.

CHECK IT OUT

Like everything else, cosmetic dentistry isn't perfect, and it may not be for everyone. But in most cases, it can make an enormous difference in how your teeth look, so it's certainly worth looking into. It's not possible to cover all the newest brands of bleaching agents and bleaching systems here, and there will be new ones appearing after this book is published, but we'll be keeping you up-to-date on cosmetic dentistry (and in more detail) in *The Tooth Fitness Digest*.

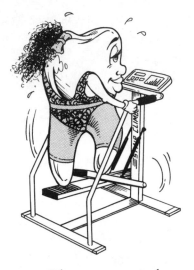

Chapter 14

Restorations

After your hygiene therapy, the dentist will present his treatment plans and you must decide which one is best for you. The information presented in this chapter is intended to help you understand what the dentist is talking about so you won't be intimidated by the choices. You'll be introduced to a wide array of dental restorations: amalgams, composites, gold, porcelain-to-metal, as well as partial dentures and dentures. A book can't see, and it can't tell you what type of restoration you'll need (that decision will be up to you and your dentist), but with a basic understanding of the available restorative materials, you'll be able to make an educated decision.

KEY TERMS

Before you try to understand anything else, you should understand the terminology universally used by dentists when discussing your repair options.

Restoration In dental lingo, a *restoration* refers to any material or device (fixed or removable) that is used (1) to replace lost tooth structure and restore the tooth to function or (2) to replace a lost tooth. There are many types of restorations, including fillings, crowns, bridges, partial dentures, and full dentures, all of which will be discussed later in the chapter.

Filling A *filling* usually refers to a restoration that restores part of a tooth. Types of fillings include amalgams, composites, inlays, onlays, gold foils, and temporary fillings.

Crown A *crown* is a restoration that restores all the tooth's crown (the portion of the tooth above the gum line that is covered by enamel).

Bridge A *bridge* is a nonremovable restoration used to replace one or more lost teeth.

Appliance This term refers to any removable restoration.

Partial denture A *partial denture* is a removable appliance used to replace lost teeth.

Denture A *denture* is a removable appliance used to replace the loss of either all the upper teeth, all the lowers, or both.

Cavity In dental terminology a *cavity* does not mean "decay," even though most people use the term that way. Actually, a cavity is what you have after the decay has been removed. When the dentist prepares your tooth for a restoration, he not only removes all the decay but also enlarges the resulting cavity. He does this in order to accomplish several things: to allow the filling material to be inserted, to ensure that there will be healthy dentin underneath the enamel, and to position the margin (edge) of the filling in an area that can easily be reached by the toothbrush.

Taking an impression This is a method of creating a model of a tooth (or teeth) and/or all or any part of the jaw. The model, usually of plaster or hard dental stone, is used in the process of making inlays, onlays, bridges, partials, and dentures, and for study models (which the dentist uses as a diagnostic tool).

Other terminology When describing or explaining a procedure, your dentist is likely to use other terms besides those listed here. Many of them will be found in the Glossary, but if he uses one you're not familiar with, ask him explain it to you.

CLASSIFYING FILLINGS

Dentists have standard ways of classifying fillings according to location. First, for simplicity, the tooth is divided into sections:

1. The top (*occlusal*)

2. The front (*buccal,* if it's the front part of the back teeth; and *labial,* if it's the front part of the front teeth)

3. The back (*lingual*), facing the tongue

4. The side facing the tonsils (*distal*)

5. The side facing the lips (*mesial*)

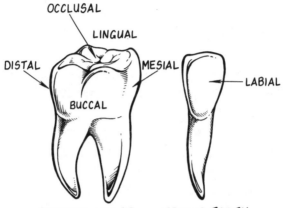

SECOND MOLAR   FRONT TOOTH

The type of filling is then designated by abbreviation:

1. O (occlusal) when a filling involves just the top of the tooth

2. B (buccal) if it fills a cavity on the side facing the cheeks

3. L (lingual) if it involves the side toward the tongue

4. DO (distal occlusal), if it involves the top and the side of the tooth facing the tonsils

5. MO (mesial occlusal), if it concerns the top and the side of the tooth facing the lips

6. MOD (mesial-occlusal-distal), if it involves the top and two sides

7. MODL (mesial-occlusal-distal-lingual), if it involves the top, the two sides, and the back

8. MODB (mesial-occulsal-distal-buccal), when it involves the top, two sides, and the front

9. MODBL, when all five surfaces are involved

FILLING LOCATIONS

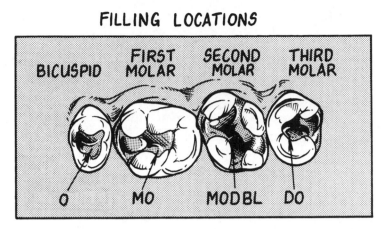

I know what you're thinking: "This isn't simple, it's confusing! Why can't they just call them front, back, and so forth?" Well, this terminology may be confusing for you at first glance, but it makes it easier for dentists to communicate with each other. It's much easier to say "distal" than to say "the side of the tooth facing toward the back of the mouth." This is one of those situations where a picture or two is worth at least a few thousand words.

Now at least you'll know what he's talking about if your dentist uses "dental-eze" to describe the location of the filling you need or if your insurance forms use these designations. By the way, you should also know that every time a letter is added, the cost of the filling goes up, regardless of what type of filling material is used. Thus, an MODBL filling could be three to four times more expensive than an O one.

FILLING MATERIALS

A number of very good filling materials are available these days. New materials and improvements on the old ones are being introduced all the time. In just about every case, there'll be the right filling material for that particular job. Price is usually the only obstacle to getting the best filling possible. But if you can't afford the very best, there will always be a less expensive choice that will do the job until you can. When your dentist presents you with the best treatment plan he can put together, it will include the most appropriate filling for your individual situation. But the final choice will be up to you.

Amalgam

The *amalgam* (or silver, or silver-mercury) filling starts out as a powdered mixture of silver (33 to 37 percent), tin (12 to 14 percent), copper (0 to 3 percent), and zinc (0 to 1 percent). Liquid mercury (about 50 percent) is then added to mix and bind the other metals together to form a paste (in the same way as water is used to blend the ingredients of a cake mix) that can be easily placed into the cavity. Some, but not all, of the mercury is squeezed out before the paste is placed into the cavity. After the paste is placed in the cavity, it is "carved" to conform to the contours of the tooth, and the resultant filling, which partially sets in a few minutes, can be chewed on in a few hours.

Without the support of enough tooth structure, an amalgam filling isn't strong enough to withstand the forces of chewing. Therefore they are least effective when placed in large cavities. If the decay is extensive and undermines the cusps of the tooth, an onlay or crown must be used. On the other hand, amalgam is easy and quick to work with and it's inexpensive. If it weren't for the controversy over mercury it would unquestionably be considered a great filling material. The pros and cons of having a filling that contains mercury placed in your teeth are discussed in Chapter 18, "Fluoride and Mercury."

Composite

Composite veneers for the front teeth are discussed in the chapter on cosmetic dentistry (Chapter 13). But composites are used as filling material as well. In fact, advances in this tooth-colored material have made it more versatile than ever. Today's composites not only adhere to the tooth better but also resist temperature changes. Some contain materials that resist decay. There's even a composite that can withstand the forces of mastication. And composites are the most natural-looking fillings. These improvements mean that composites can often be used in place of amalgam fillings if you're concerned about aesthetics or the mercury in amalgam fillings.

The important thing is to make sure that your dentist is up-to-date on the latest composite materials. My personal recommendation is to use composite fillings whenever possible and to use gold, or porcelain-to-metal crowns, if the decay is so extensive that composites can't be used. If you have children, I suggest composite fillings rather than amalgams, but let your pediatric dentist explain your filling options before you make a decision.

Gold

With a few exceptions, gold is the best restorative material. Its limitations have nothing to do with how good it is but with cost and aesthetics. If you can afford it and are comfortable with how it looks, then I suggest you use it in every case where a composite or amalgam is not the material of choice. I don't recommend gold for baby teeth.

Inlays Inlays are custom-made cast gold restorations that can be used in many of the same types of cavities in which amalgams and composites are used. Inlays don't break down like amalgams and composites, and they wear at the same rate as the tooth. They can be used instead of, or to replace, amalgams if you're concerned about mercury, or instead of composites if you're concerned with durability and longevity. They last a long time, twenty years or more if you take care of them, but are also more expensive.

Onlays When you hear this term, you know that decay has progressed too far for a tooth to be restored by an amalgam or composite filling, or even an inlay. Onlays, like inlays, are cast gold but, as the name implies, they extend *over* the tooth's cusps. When a tooth's cusp has been broken off, or when decay under the cusps has progressed to such a degree that they no longer support the forces of mastication, an onlay (or a crown) is used. Because of the protection onlays give the cusps, onlays are more commonly used than are inlays. They are usually less expensive than crowns.

Gold foil At one time gold foil was the filling of choice for decay between the front teeth and at the gum line. Applying this material is an arduous and time-consuming process. It also subjects the tooth to a great deal of trauma because the dentist has to pound on it with a device that is like a miniature jackhammer in order to insert the gold foil in the cavity. With the advent of composites it's rarely used anymore. Other than the skill it takes to insert them I can't find anything good to say about them. I'd never have one done on my teeth, and needless to say, I don't recommend them.

Temporary

This is an easy one to describe. A temporary filling is one that is used to temporarily fill a cavity until a permanent restoration can be placed. It's often used in emergency situations, or when there's not enough time to put in a permanent restoration. Also, because it often contains a nerve-calming ingredient, a temporary filling is placed when the decay has progressed too close to the nerve. This gives the nerve a chance to calm down so a restoration can eventually be placed.

CROWNS AND BRIDGES

In addition to fillings, there are other types of restorations used to repair your teeth and to replace those that are missing.

Crowns

A *crown* is a restoration that covers the entire tooth surface. It is used when so much tooth is lost that no filling will provide the strength and protection needed to allow it to continue functioning as it should. To place a crown, the tooth must be reduced enough to allow the crown to fit around the tooth and to allow for enough thickness on the crown's chewing surface so that as it wears down it won't expose the tooth under it. A crown can be made of gold, porcelain-to-metal, porcelain, or acrylic. When placed on the front teeth, it's more commonly called a *cap* or a *jacket*. A crown is often needed to cover a tooth that has had a root canal (see pages 221–23), because when the nerves and blood supply have been removed the tooth dries out and is much more susceptible to fracturing.

Gold crown A gold crown can be placed on any tooth, but because it isn't the most aesthetically appealing of restorations, it is usually used on the back teeth. Gold crowns cost about the same as most porcelain-to-metal crowns.

Porcelain-to-metal crown Porcelain bonded to a metal alloy at a high temperature is now the material of choice when a tooth, front or back, must be crowned and aesthetics is a concern. In the past, pure porcelain crowns were used for the front teeth, and gold was used for the back teeth. Porcelain alone gives a beautiful finish, but is not strong enough to withstand the chewing forces to which the back teeth are subjected. Gold crowns can withstand all the chewing forces, but while it's considered very beautiful as a ring or necklace, by most standards it's not considered beautiful when it can be seen glinting from your mouth.

Porcelain fused to metal combines the best qualities of each material to make a filling that is both strong and visually pleasing. For the back teeth, the best and longest-lasting design is a crown with a metal chewing surface and a porcelain front (or *facing*). Although some people don't want any metal showing at all, the use of porcelain on the chewing surface has its drawbacks. It can fracture from the metal base, and, even though it looks smooth, it's abrasive enough to wear down the opposing natural tooth at a faster rate than metal does. In most cases, for the front teeth, porcelain without the metal backing can be used to cover the entire surface because the forces placed upon the front teeth aren't as great as on the back teeth.

There are many variations on the porcelain-to-metal restoration, and new materials appear regularly. So if you're concerned about aesthetics ask your dentist which material would be best in your case.

Bridges

A *bridge* is a fixed restoration of cast gold or porcelain-to-metal that is used to permanently replace lost teeth. When done correctly and cemented to the natural teeth, it's extremely difficult to remove. I like this term because it refers to what this restoration actually does—bridges the gap left by a missing tooth or missing teeth.

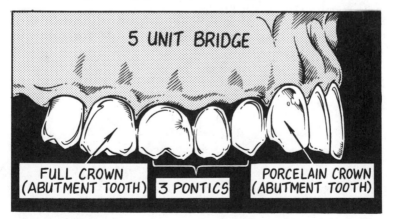

5 UNIT BRIDGE

FULL CROWN (ABUTMENT TOOTH)   3 PONTICS   PORCELAIN CROWN (ABUTMENT TOOTH)

There are many kinds of bridges. There are some that attach to one tooth and hang over, called *cantilever bridges*, ones that attach to two teeth, and those that attach to more than two teeth.

If you need a bridge it means the dentist will have to place crowns on the natural teeth adjacent to the lost one(s)—even if they aren't decayed—in order to attach the bridge. If you're replacing one missing tooth it means that two teeth will have to be crowned and a replacement false tooth attached between the two crowns. It's sometimes necessary to crown more than two natural teeth to support the bridge: when it's a long span (replacing many teeth) or when too much bone has been lost around the adjacent tooth for it to adequately withstand the chewing stresses placed upon the bridge. The teeth that are crowned to support a bridge (or partial denture) are called *abutment* teeth. The replacement tooth (or "false tooth") is called a *pontic* and is either gold or porcelain bonded to metal.

Each member of the bridge, including the abutment teeth and the pontic, is referred to as a "unit." Thus, if one missing tooth is replaced, the bridge is referred to as a three-unit bridge. As you move up the ladder of lost teeth the cost will increase with each additional unit: a four-unit bridge will be more expensive than a three-unit bridge, and so on.

Given apples for apples, a fixed bridge is always better than a removable appliance, such as a partial denture, because it's more aesthetic, provides more function, and is less stressful on the abutment teeth.

DENTAL APPLIANCES

The term *appliance* usually refers to dental "hardware" that is not permanently attached, such as the partial denture and the full denture.

Partial Dentures

A partial denture, commonly just referred to as a "partial," is a removable appliance used to replace missing teeth. Along with implants (discussed in Chapter 15), it's the only choice left if you've lost all the back teeth on either or both sides of your jaw, upper or lower. Also, a partial can be used to replace missing teeth if you can't afford a bridge. The main differences between a fixed bridge and a removable partial are:

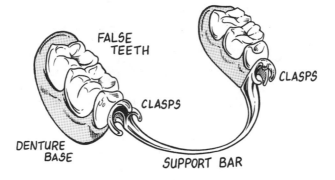

FALSE TEETH

CLASPS

CLASPS

DENTURE BASE

SUPPORT BAR

PARTIAL DENTURE

- ☐ *The price*. If the same number of teeth are involved, partials generally will be less expensive.

- ☐ *Performance*. Partials are removable; bridges aren't. The partial is attached by clasps to the abutment teeth. In some cases, if the natural teeth aren't the right shape to properly hold the clasps, the abutment teeth must be crowned. If the partial doesn't have a back tooth to support the replacement teeth, it must rely on the abutment tooth and the saddlelike denture base (which holds the false teeth in place and sits on the jawbone to provide support while chewing). Therefore the partial is not as strong as a bridge, places more stress on the abutment teeth, and is less efficient for chewing than a fixed bridge.

- ☐ *Durability*. If they are both made correctly and you maintain them, a bridge will usually last much longer than a partial.

- ☐ *Aesthetics.* Even the best-made partial denture isn't as appealing as a bridge. The clasps usually show, and the place where the denture base overlaps the jawbone ridge can be unsightly.

- ☐ *Maintenance.* The partial denture is easier to clean than a bridge because it can be removed. But the denture base will periodically have to be *relined* (new material added to the underside of the denture base) and the clasps adjusted to keep the proper fit.

Your dentist will know whether a bridge or a partial appliance is best for your situation. If your dentist thinks a bridge is the best choice, but you're partial to a partial just because it's less expensive, you should choose the bridge . . . you'll be a lot happier and end up spending less money over the long haul.

Full Dentures

The full denture is discussed in the next chapter, "Dentures and Implants."

HOW LONG DO THEY LAST?

The amount of time any restoration will last will depend on a few different factors:

☐ Whether it was the best restoration for that particular situation in the first place (if you choose an amalgam when a crown is recommended, the amalgam won't last as long as it would doing a job it's better suited for)

☐ How well it was made (millions of fillings fail because of poor workmanship)

☐ Your diet and chewing habits (grinders and clenchers are harder on restorations)

☐ How well you take care of it (many fillings have to be redone because of new decay caused by poor oral hygiene)

Thus, if you select a good dentist, choose the best restoration for the job, and take care of it, you can vastly extend the life of any restoration, from a composite to a denture. When you make your choice of a treatment plan make sure your dentist explains the trade-offs between cost and durability for the restorations you're considering.

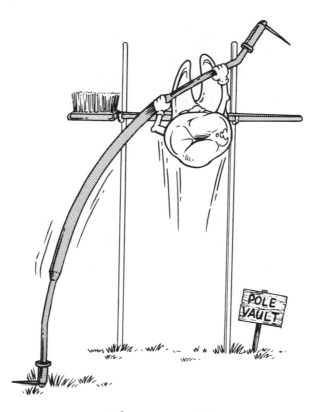

Chapter 15

Dentures and Implants

If you happen to be one of the over 13 million people who have lost all your teeth, the term *prevention* won't have the same meaning for you as it does for the rest of the population. But even though it's too late for you to save your teeth, there's a lot you can do to make the best of a difficult situation. You can take advantage of the latest in denture and implant technology. Not only can dentures be made better than ever before, but *implants* (devices implanted into the jawbone to which an artificial tooth, bridge, partial, or denture can be attached) have dramatically improved the options available for those who have lost their teeth.

But before I get into what you can do for yourself, I'm going to tell you how you can help prevent what happened to you from happening to those you care about. "But what could I possibly do?" you may be thinking. "After all, I'm not a dentist and I didn't do such a good job of keeping my own teeth." Well, you'd be surprised . . . You can play a very important role in getting the preventive message out to others—your children, your grandchildren, nieces, nephews, or anyone else you care enough about to make a positive difference in their oral and general health.

WHAT YOU CAN DO FOR OTHERS

People sometimes get discouraged trying to fight dental disease and think that dentures are the best way to deal with it: "Well, if I didn't have any teeth I wouldn't have any problems with them." But you know that giving up your natural teeth for dentures is like exchanging a small can of worms for a huge can of worms. In fact, you're the *only* one who can tell these people what it's really like to lose your teeth. Only you know the aesthetic and social problems associated with dentures. Only you know the way dentures can affect what you eat. Only you know how much money you have to spend on denture creams, adhesives, and having relines and new dentures made. In short, only you can tell them about what you've had to go through because you never had access to information about prevention.

Don't be embarrassed or feel guilty; tell them the truth. All the denture patients I know have denture horror stories they're embarrassed to talk about. I'm sure you have a few of your own, and that's exactly what I want you to relay to your loved ones. Because of your experience, you'll be able to reach them with a vivid message impossible to convey in a book. Not only will you be the one who provides them with valuable information but, more important, you'll become a source of motivation for them.

I'm not suggesting you take on the responsibility for their dental health, nor should you try to force them into anything. You don't have to be pushy (that approach usually won't work anyway); just the facts will do fine. In short, you can't make them drink the water, but you can sure show them the way to the well. Some of your friends and family may not have heard of *Tooth Fitness*. If they haven't, you can give them a gift of the book, or at least tell them about it.

I know you understand what I'm asking you to do. The message you're bringing will be powerful and effective because it's coming from someone they know. I'm going to thank you ahead of time, not for me, but for them.

DENTURES

What You Can Do for Yourself

A *full denture* is a removable appliance used to replace the loss of all teeth, either all the uppers, all the lowers, or both. A *partial denture*, as its name implies, is used when there are still teeth remaining for the denture to attach to. Dentures are usually made of an acrylic base (George Washington's denture base was made of wood) with either porcelain or plastic teeth. Since making any old denture is easy, but making a good denture is a complicated procedure and requires skill and experience, the single most important thing you can do for yourself is to find a good denture specialist. In the trade, he's called a prosthodontist (see pages 224–25). If there is no prosthodontist available in your vicinity, look for a general dentist who specializes in making dentures.

The act of chewing is very complicated, and making dentures that allow you to correctly perform this intricate process should not be left to "short-order denture cooks." (There may be an exceptional good one, but you usually end up getting what you pay for.) Far too many denture wearers are so used to cut-rate, assembly-line dentures that they find it difficult to understand that the difference between a poorly made denture and a well-made denture is like the difference between night and day.

Moreover, because of all the improvements to denture making you can't afford to trust your dentures to someone who's still making them the way he did twenty or even ten years ago. Having a specialist make your dentures means he'll be versed in the newest techniques and materials, such as overlay dentures (which are a type of partial denture attached to the remaining teeth) and the grafting of materials to the jawbone ridge (if the ridge has been worn away too much to hold a regular denture).

Until you've actually had a well-made denture you won't know how much difference it can make—to your appearance, to how and what you can eat, and to your overall health. A good set of dentures is more than worth the additional cost and the extra time spent having them made because they'll function better, last longer, and prevent the loss of bone from your jaw's ridges. Poorly made dentures are the main cause of such bone loss. If you don't get good dentures, especially if they're your first set, you may end up not having have enough jawbone left to have dentures made in the future. This is not a place to pinch the penny.

How to Find a Denture Expert

Chapter 6 describes in detail how to go about finding a qualified dentist and hygienist. The same principles apply here except you'll be seeking a prosthodontist or a dentist who specializes in dentures. Keep in mind that a personal recommendation is always the most reliable.

After you've obtained a promising recommendation, call and ask for a short consultation visit. The consultation visit is the time to ask the dentist a few key questions to see if he's the one you want to do the work. Here's what to ask:

1. How much experience have you had making dentures?

2. If it turns out, upon examination, that my condition is beyond your talents, will you refer me to a dentist who can handle my case?

3. Will you present me with a plan for the best possible treatment, along with alternatives?

4. How long can the denture be expected to last?

5. Will the dentures affect my tasting ability? And is there anything that can be done to help?

6. What are the pro's and con's of having a backup set made?

Getting Down to Business

Now that you've definitely decided to go ahead with a particular denture specialist, you need to realize that having dentures made is a two-way street. For his part, the dentist will listen to your story and speak to your concerns and questions. Then he'll tell you what type of denture you need and give you a number of choices based on quality and your ability to pay. Now you must be willing to do your part, which means trusting his judgment, following his instructions, and allowing him to do his job. It also means making sure you understand what he's doing and why. Some of the questions that might come up for you include:

1. How can the dentures be made to look as natural as possible? Have your dentist explain the difference between porcelain and plastic teeth and about adjusting the color to match your age and complexion. Ask him about varying the sizes, shapes, and positions of the teeth to make them look more natural. Can he add pigment to the acrylic denture base to match the color of your gums? You can also ask him about placing a filling or two in the back teeth—this really fools people who think they can spot a denture.

2. Should I wear them at night?

3. What is the best way to keep them clean?

4. How often should I have checkups?

5. What is the best way to deal with sore spots?

6. How often should I have my dentures relined? This will vary from denture wearer to denture wearer, so follow his advice.

7. What about over-the-counter denture adhesives, denture creams, and at-home reline procedures? I don't recommend them, except in emergency situations, because if you have a frequent need for them you need a denture checkup and probably a professional reline or even a new denture. Tens of millions of dollars are spent each year on adhesives, pseudorelines, and denture creams. If dentures were made right in the first place and relined when necessary, this wouldn't be the case, and you'd save all the money you spend on patchwork home treatment.

8. What are the best ways to adjust to new dentures?

Chances are your denture dentist won't judge you by the denture you wore to his office, no matter how poorly it was made, or now fits, because he'll know you were unlucky in selecting your previous denture maker. But to make sure he doesn't jump to any conclusions, tell him clearly that you've seen the light and want the best denture he can make and that you'll take care of your end. If you absolutely can't afford the best, take the best you can afford. But remember, in the long run you'll be paying more because you'll end up having your denture remade more often.

Denture Nutrition

No matter what choice of dentures you make, understand that dentures will affect your nutrition because even the best of them lack the chewing efficiency of your natural teeth. Therefore you *must* compensate nutritionally.

Poorly made dentures, or those that haven't been relined when the should be, may only be 15 to 30 percent as efficient as natural teeth. As a result, many denture wearers adjust their diet to fit their dentures and end up only eating foods that are easy to chew with dentures—at the expense of eating what they should. This diet—which I call "the denture food diet"—is characterized by the elimination of many raw fruits, vegetables, and grains in favor of re-fined, processed, soft, and overcooked foods that are devoid of fiber, vitamins, and other nutrients. Not only does this diet play havoc with your digestive system but it affects your overall health as well. Your health simply can't afford ill-fitting dentures. I'll give you the same message I've given all the denture patients I've consulted with—you've got to be more conscious of your nutritional needs than when you had your natural teeth. (The next chapter, "Nutrition and Your Teeth," will delve into this area more deeply.)

Denture wearers tend to suffer from all kinds of health problems, not the least of which are digestive in nature, like intestinal disorders, constipation, and hemorrhoids. I've spoken with hundreds of denture wearers, and every one of them told me that their health seemed to deteriorate after they got their dentures. If you do nothing else to help balance the loss of chewing efficiency, make sure you take a good multiple vitamin and mineral supplement and add fiber to your diet. Many kinds of fiber additives are available, but I think psyllium husks are the best of the lot. The brand I use is Yerba Prima. It can be found in health food stores. Avoid any brand that contains sugar.

If your dentures make it impossible to chew raw foods, I strongly suggest you grate your vegetables or lightly steam them. You won't have to chew as much, and if you don't overcook them you'll still get the nutritional value they contain. Drinking raw vegetable and fruit juices is another excellent way to get these vital nutrients. Most health food stores carry an assortment of great juicers (or can order them), and most have nutritional consultants who'll be more than happy to help you make choices about diet, fiber, vitamins, and other supplements that can help keep you healthy—even if you're a denture wearer.

Make sure to tell your physician that you're wearing dentures, and let him know what you're eating. I believe that if the medical profession paid more attention to the total patient and took into account his or her oral condition, they'd find that many problems are the direct result of nutritional deficiencies caused by the inability to chew properly.

What happened to your natural teeth is water under the bridge. Now you must move on and do the best you can with what you have. Get the best denture you can, make sure you compensate for the nutritional deficiencies that stem from wearing dentures,

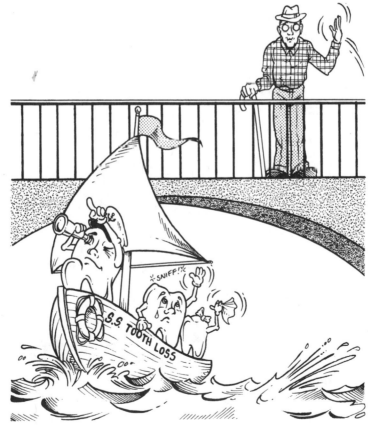

and do what you can to spread the preventive message to your friends and loved ones.

IMPLANTS

Implants, introduced in the early eighties, are now the hottest of the dental technologies. They can be used to replace a single missing tooth or a whole set of teeth. Implants are specially designed pieces of metal or ceramic material that are surgically implanted into the jawbone. In time bone forms around them and they are firmly held in the jaw, much like the roots of natural teeth, except that they don't have the periodontal ligament to cushion the impact of chewing. The portion that protrudes through your gums can be crowned or used as an abutment for attaching bridges or dentures and partials. If you're interested in the types of metals and techniques that are used, or any other detailed information, your dentist will be able to provide it to you.

The success ratio of any type of implant increases if there are natural teeth to help withstand and evenly distribute the chewing forces. For example, if implants alone were used to anchor a full denture they would be taking a bigger load than if you had ten natural teeth to help them out. So if you are contemplating implants, saving as many healthy teeth as you can will be very important. Don't have any teeth pulled until you consult with your implant dentist.

The Implant Expert

The placement of implants is complicated. Dentists need a lot of training, experience, and skill to be qualified in this field. For an implant to be successful it not only must be properly inserted but also requires a dedicated effort, on the part of the patient, to keep it clean and disease-free.

Implant technology is improving almost daily, and the only way to ensure that you're getting the best treatment is to find the best dentist and ask the best questions. People sometimes resist the time and effort it takes to do this, but if you're serious about having this procedure done it's really the only way. Start by using the suggestions in "Finding a Dentist and a Dental Hygienist," Chapter 6. Dental schools are on the cutting edge of implant technology, so if a dental school is available to you it'll be a great place to have implants done. Once you think you've found a good implant specialist (a qualified dentist, prosthodontist, or oral surgeon) I suggest you first schedule a consultation with him. (Some dentists don't charge for this, but be sure to ask.) It'll give you time to ask your questions and, more important, to ask him to detail his qualifications before you decide to use him. Here's what you should ask:

1. Have you had any special training for implants? How much? Don't just take his word for it—ask to see any diplomas or certificates he has.

2. How long have you been doing implants? How many have you done? (The more he has done the better.) How much of your practice is devoted to them?

3. Do you have photographs and testimonials from patients you've treated?

4. How long can I expect the implants to last?

5. How do I go about caring for them? If you neglected to take care of your real teeth, you won't be able to get away with that approach now. Implants take much more care than natural teeth, and if you don't take care of them they will not last. Make sure you religiously adhere to your dentist's follow-up instructions and show up for the recall appointments. You should diligently follow the home-care procedures in Chapter 5 and work closely with your hygienist, because along with occlusal stress, the number one cause of implant failure is poor oral hygiene.

If you're unclear about any implant procedure the dentist suggests, are unsure about his abilities, or don't have confidence in him, then seek a second opinion. If everything checks out with the second opinion, I guarantee you'll feel more confident and it will have been worth the extra effort. And if it doesn't, you can switch dentists before any harm is done.

When Should They Be Done?

In many cases people are unable to wear conventional dentures because the jawbone ridge cannot retain them. Also, some dentures wearers are unhappy with how dentures look. But now, thanks to implants, dentures are no longer the last resort. Implants not only offer another option, but for many people may be the only choice left. Besides, unlike dentures, they won't fall out at inappropriate times, like when you're eating or making love.

Implants can also be used to replace a single lost tooth or several teeth if you don't want a bridge because you'd rather not crown healthy teeth. They can be used, too, to provide additional support for bridges and partial dentures.

Because placing implants is still an emerging dental science it's a relatively expensive procedure. For most people who need to replace teeth, the question of whether to use implants usually comes down to economics rather than whether they are the treatment of choice. As I've said before (once or twice or a hundred times), you can't afford to use cost as the only criterion for having the best possible dental work done. If your choice is between teeth or no teeth, choose teeth—even if they are artificially implanted ones. Ultimately it's a matter of health. If you can't properly chew the foods you need to keep you healthy, you're not only diminishing the quality of your life but shortening your life expectancy. Look at it this way: it may seem like a lot of money now, but if it helps you live longer and improves the quality of your life, how can you not afford it?

We'll keep you up-to-date on the newest innovations in denture and implant technology in *The Tooth Fitness Digest*.

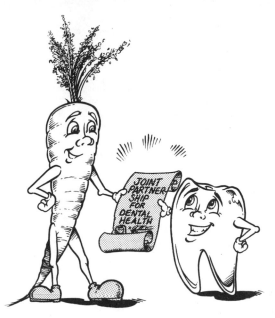

Chapter 16

Nutrition and Your Teeth

Although it's possible to eat an unhealthy diet and still prevent dental disease, you can do so only if you strictly (and I do mean strictly) follow the procedures outlined in the home care chapter (Chapter 5), spend extra time with the toothbrush and other preventive tools, and establish a permanent relationship with your hygienist and dentist. This is the only way you can compensate for a poor diet and ward off what could be prevented easily and naturally by a healthy diet.

The amount of time you must spend taking care of your teeth and gums will be directly proportional to how unhealthy your diet is, especially if you're decay-prone and have, or have had, gum disease. (Eat better, spend less time; eat worse, spend more time.) If you're willing to spend the extra time, you don't have to care, or even know, about nutrition in relationship to dental health. But just because you can, with a great deal of effort, keep your teeth and gums healthy while eating a disease-causing diet doesn't mean the rest of your body will be so fortunate. Wouldn't you suspect that if an unhealthy diet promotes dental disease, it might promote other diseases as well? In fact, that's precisely the case.

DEGENERATIVE DISEASE AND DIET

Dental disease is the most prevalent disease not only in the United States, but in the world. According to the guidelines used to classify disease, it's actually an epidemic, although I can't figure out why it isn't treated as one.

Dental disease is also classified as a degenerative disease. In general terms degenerative disease is the deterioration of a tissue or organ in which normal function or structure is impaired. In dental disease it's the gums and teeth that deteriorate until both function and structure are impaired. In my opinion, most degenerative disease is diet-related. When, over a long period of time, the nutrients needed by the body to maintain health and resist disease are unavailable in sufficient quantities, or the body is subjected to excessive amounts of harmful substances, degenerative disease develops. Scurvy, caused by lack of vitamin C, and kwashiorkor, which results from prolonged protein deficiency, are two examples of degenerative diseases caused by insufficient nutrition. Prolonged and excessive use of alcohol, tobacco, or foods high in saturated fats and cholesterol contributes to liver disease, cancer, and heart disease, which are just a few examples of degenerative disease caused by harmful substances. As the body is depleted of vital nutrients and stressed trying to rid itself of harmful substances, it becomes vulnerable to diseases that a healthy body could normally resist.

A bad diet gets you coming and going. It affects you as it enters your body (dental disease), while it's going through the body (digestive disease, cancer, liver and heart disease), and on its way out (hemorrhoids and constipation). Therefore if you don't eat a healthy diet, not only are you putting your teeth and gums at risk for dental disease, you're putting the rest of you at risk for even worse trouble.

The wheels should be turning now . . . with a little thought you can see that diet, dental disease, and other degenerative diseases are connected. A dedicated oral hygiene program can prevent dental disease, but if you continue to eat a disease-causing diet, the rest of your body will pay a heavy, even fatal, price for your inattention to nature's nutritional laws.

It would take an entire book to show you how important nutrition is to your health and well-being. Since I can't provide all of this information in one chapter, I'll tell you where to find it. At the end of the chapter you'll see a list of my favorite books on nutrition. The best place to look for these books is at your local health food store. Some health food stores also have certified nutritional counselors who can help you decide which books and health products would be of value for your particular situation, answer your questions about nutrition, and get you started on your quest for better health. Becoming more involved with good nutrition means you'll be practicing true preventive medicine. It will not only make caring for your teeth easier but will enhance the quality of your life and extend your life expectancy.

The type of diet most Americans consider healthy is vastly different from what our ancestors ate. A quick look back in time will help you understand why "progress" is not always synonymous with "health."

Looking Back

For millions of years human beings ate a balanced and natural diet. In fact, as recently as sixty years ago there were still tribes of people, in different parts of the world, whose diets were uncontaminated by our so-called civilized food (refined, processed, preserved, and overly cooked). Their diet remained basically the same as it has been for tens of thousands of years. These people were in excellent health, and their mouths were virtually free of dental disease. This diet, even though it varied from place to place and evolved without the help of nutritionists, included all the nutrients, vitamins, and minerals needed to prevent degenerative disease.

But picture what would have happened to our ancestors if they had given up their natural diet and adopted our modern diet—but without the benefits of modern dentistry and medicine. Decay would be as rampant as it is today—but they couldn't go to a hygienist for cleaning, hygiene instruction, and guidance; couldn't go to a dentist to have their pain relieved or their teeth repaired. The affected teeth would continue to decay and would eventually rot away. The teeth that weren't lost to decay would soon fall prey to gum disease, because they wouldn't know how to prevent gum disease anymore than how to prevent decay. They wouldn't have the luxury of being able to have false teeth either. And even if they did have false teeth, they couldn't go to the supermarket and buy the cooked and processed foods that today's denture wearers must eat. Nor could they go to the health food store and buy vitamins to replace what they weren't getting from their diet.

Suffering from constant gum disease and deprived of the nutrients the body's immune system needs to fight this and other diseases, their general health would deteriorate. As the body's defenses weakened, they would be subjected to all kinds of infections, and, at some point, heart disease and cancer would make short work of them —as if they didn't have enough trouble dealing with wild animals.

In short, had our early ancestors eaten what most people eat today and suffered from the degenerative diseases we now suffer from, humankind simply wouldn't have survived. (In *Nutrition and Physical Degeneration*, one of the books on my list, the author brilliantly documents the negative results of introducing a modern diet to so-called primitive people—I highly recommend you read it.)

Yet the diet that would have cut short humankind's existence on the planet is the same diet that people today generally believe is fine and dandy. But just because we have doctors and dentists to treat the many diseases caused by poor nutrition doesn't mean we can get away with abusing our bodies, any more than our ancestors could have.

This isn't just theory. Nature's laws don't change. The only way we've been able to survive the harmful changes in our diet is because we have the knowledge and technology to treat some of the life-threatening side effects that result from such a diet. But just because we can sometimes manage to keep people alive longer doesn't mean we are nutritionally evolved and in no way means that we understand the concept of prevention. Think about this for a moment. Our ancestors had no toothbrush, no toothpaste, no floss, no water irrigation device, and no mouthwash. Their preventive tools consisted of twigs and pieces of bone—and their natural diet. That was enough for them to keep dental disease at bay. Today, even with all our modern dental tools, not to mention the hygienist and dentist, dental disease is epidemic. Why? I'll say it again: we've changed from a natural, disease-preventing diet to an unnatural, disease-causing one.

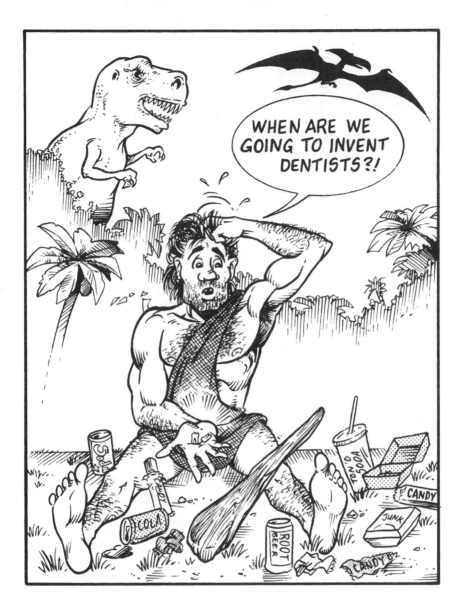

When you consider the many diseases we are confronted with—dental disease, cancer, heart disease, etc.—you have to admit we're not exactly winning the war against degenerative disease. I'm not suggesting you run out and get a loincloth and spear and find a nice dry cave to live in. You don't have to live the way our ancestors did to be as healthy as they were. But you do have to pay attention to your diet.

THE BEST DIET FOR YOUR TEETH

The most important thing you must do if you want to use your diet as a preventive dental tool is to make a firm decision to change your diet from an unhealthy one to a healthy one. This means you should increase your intake of fruits, vegetables (raw or lightly steamed), grains (rice, wheat, millet, etc.), seeds, and nuts; eliminate all refined sugars (as you'll see, much of the sugar you get is in the form of "hidden" sugars); and cut out as much processed, preserved, overly cooked, soft, and sticky foods as possible.

You'll also need to make sure that whatever you put into your mouth is fully masticated and that all "leftovers" are removed from your mouth as soon after eating as possible, especially if they contain sugar. In other words, eat well, chew well, and clean your teeth. If you can't brush after a meal containing soft or refined foods, finish off the meal with firm, fibrous raw foods—like apples and carrots. If you can't do that, rinse with water or chew sugar-free gum.

If for some reason you find it impossible to make the necessary dietary changes, you should at least take vitamin supplements. Read Earl Mindell's book on vitamins (see book list)—if that doesn't convince you of the need for vitamin supplements I don't think anything will. Once you establish a good vitamin program, I suggest you commit to it for at least six months and then see if you notice any difference. Don't look for overnight miracles, because you could have a long-standing deficiency and it will take a while to get your body's vitamin levels up to speed. And if you already have a health problem don't avoid medical treatment because you think vitamins alone might cure it.

I'll let Dr. Mindell's book explain the A to Z of vitamins, what they do, how they do it, what to take, and when. But I want you to know about some specific vitamins that are especially important to your oral health.

Specific Vitamins for the Teeth and Gums

While I believe a long-standing vitamin or mineral deficiency will ultimately lower your body's resistance and its ability to fight off any disease, there are some vitamin deficiencies that are more immediately connected to dental disease.

Vitamin C Although it's not true that gum disease is actually caused by a vitamin C deficiency, a long-standing deficiency increases the gum's susceptibility to infection, increases the probability of bleeding, and slows down the healing process. In effect, it makes whatever gum disease you have worse and more difficult to cure. With the more serious form of gum disease, periodontal disease, a severe deficiency of vitamin C increases the bleeding and swelling in the periodontal ligament and accelerates the destructive effects of inflammation on bone.

Vitamin A In the presence of periodontal disease, vitamin A deficiency retards the healing of infection, increases the pocket depth, accelerates the formation of subgingival calculus, and in general makes your gum disease more difficult to heal. Lack of vitamin A has also been associated with abnormal bone and tooth formation and an increase in leukoplakia.

Vitamin B complex A deficiency of the B vitamins can increase the severity of gingivitis, including ANUG (acute necrotizing ulcerative gingivostomatitis), and cause lesions of the gums, tongue, soft tissues of the mouth, periodontal tissues, and at the junction where the upper and lower lips meet (called *angular cheilitis*, in case you were wondering about it).

If you give your body the vitamins it needs to internally fight the battle against gum disease, your oral hygiene efforts will be more effective. If you're not making the effort to keep your mouth free of germs, and you also have nutritional deficiencies, the body won't be able to handle the massive increase of bacteria. Disease will gain a stronger foothold and proceed more rapidly because both lines of defense—your oral hygiene and the body's ability to resist disease —are lowered.

SUGAR (SUCROSE)

I discussed sucrose in relation to decay in Chapter 1. Now let's look at it from a slightly different angle. The first mention of sugar in historical records was way back in 325 B.C., but until around the fifteenth century it was only available to the rich. Since then its availability to the general population has continually increased to the point where the average American will consume over one hundred pounds of it per year.

Sugar is found naturally in fruits and vegetables, ranging from a little over 1 percent in most berries, pears, and cherries to about 8 percent in citrus fruits and about 15 percent in grapes. Most vegetables contain only small amounts of sugar (the sugar beet being the exception with about 15 percent sucrose). Now you know why the sugar industry refines the sugar beet and not berries.

More than one-sixth of the calories in an average diet derives from sucrose. But of the more than one hundred pounds of sugar consumed per person, only about thirty pounds is purchased in its "straight" form for home use—for coffee, for baking, on cereal, etc. Hmmm, where do you think you get the other seventy-plus pounds? Well, you get it "hidden" in the foods you purchase. Soft drinks will provide about twenty pounds, and the remaining fifty pounds come mainly from cakes, pies, cereals, and snacks like Twinkies, but also from by candy and chewing gum, canned foods, frozen foods, and dairy products (ice cream leading the pack here). An ounce of sugar here, an ounce or two there, and before you know it, in only one year, over one hundred pounds of sugar has passed through your oral cavity.

There is no argument about what sugar can do to your teeth (see, for example, the description of a series of experiments on decay and sugar, pages 29–33). But it's also a contributor to gum disease. All else being equal, the more sugar you consume the more plaque you form. Plaque also forms in the absence of sugar, but not nearly so fast. The by-products of sugar metabolism make it easier for germs to clump together and to attach themselves to the tooth. And if that weren't bad enough, some studies suggest that high sugar consumption plays a role in kidney disease, diabetes, obesity, and heart disease. Make no mistake, sugar is a very destructive substance, and not just for your teeth and gums. It may be legal, but being legal doesn't make it any less harmful.

Hidden Sugar

Sugar is everywhere. It's found in many things you already are aware of, like candy bars, gum, soft drinks, desserts, bread, juices, canned goods, as well as in many things you've probably never even considered. I've had a number of decay-prone patients who swore they had eliminated sugar from their diets, but their teeth were still decaying. At first I thought they were trying to fool me, but as we explored this phenomenon further we found, to everyone's surprise, that they were getting significant amounts of sugar from sources they'd never suspected. Consider the following common sources of hidden sugar and see if you've been unknowingly dosing yourself with it.

Medicines Many medicines, both prescription and over-the-counter, contain sugar, most notably cough syrups and lozenges (especially cough drops). Cough syrups, liquid and tablet vitamins (especially children's vitamins), and even antibiotic syrups can contain anywhere from 10 to 75 percent sugar. Throat lozenges and cough drops may range from 50 to nearly 70 percent sugar. These medicines may not cause a serious decay problem if used only occasionally, but if you use them on a regular basis (millions of people do) they can be a major contributor. Children who have to take syrups or lozenges over long periods of time show a much higher incidence of decay than those who don't, even if there's no other source of sugar available to them. Fortunately, more and more medicines can be found that aren't sweetened with sucrose. I suggest you let your physician (who may not be aware of the sugar content of drugs) and pharmacist know that, whenever possible, you don't want sugar in your medicine.

Breath mints Ever wonder why they taste so good? Most breath mints are another source of hidden sugar. Unless they say "sugar free," half of what you are sucking on could be sugar.

Antacid tablets Another sneaky source of sugar. They range from 10 to over 50 percent sugar. Sucking on these isn't much different than sucking on candy. Tens of millions of people consume antacid tablets on a daily basis. Read the labels, ask your pharmacist for an antacid that does not contain sugar, or choose the brand that contains the least amount.

The medicine included with the sugar may be necessary, the mints enjoyable and antacid helpful but, dentally speaking, you should treat them as candy. So brush or rinse after using.

Sugar Aliases

Sugar isn't always called sugar (or sucrose). Many products that contain a lot of sucrose have exotic-sounding names that may confuse you about their content.

- [ ] **Molasses** Regardless of the brand or type of molasses, you're looking at a sucrose content of over 60 percent.

- [ ] **Turbinado** This is really only another name for sucrose, except it "only" contains 96 to 97 percent sugar instead of 99 percent. Such a deal! The remainder contains processing residues, like soil and yeasts. Don't be fooled by this one.

- [ ] **Brown sugar** Another sleeper. The only difference between brown sugar and white sugar is a small amount of molasses that gives brown sugar its color. This is almost like adding sugar to sugar.

- [ ] **Raw sugar** Just another name for turbinado sugar. Believe me, as long as they can get it, the germs that decay your teeth couldn't care less about what it's called.

- [ ] **Invert sugar** This is the name given to sucrose when it has been chemically rotated, or inverted. For all practical purposes it's sucrose—but it's about 30 percent sweeter.

- [ ] **Coupling sugar** This is a mixture of a number of types of sugars. Though it's *cariogenic* (decay causing) it's considerably less so than regular sucrose.

- [ ] **Sorghum and cane syrup** These two sweeteners are pretty much the same. Although the sugar content is less than solid sugars because not all the water is removed, they still contain significant amounts of sucrose. You should always check the label because sometimes sugar and corn syrup are added to preserve them, making them even more cariogenic.

- [ ] **Corn syrup** Although corn syrup consists mostly of sugars other than sucrose, it still must be considered cariogenic, especially for the enamel's vulnerable pits and fissures.

- [ ] **Fructose** The use of fructose as a sweetener has increased rapidly in the last fifteen years. The average person will consume over twenty pounds of fructose yearly. High-fructose corn syrup is used in many soft drinks in place of sugar. While fructose is not as cariogenic as sucrose it still must be considered cariogenic, especially when its usage is increased. Keep your eye on this one.

- ☐ **Honey** Honey is the choice of many health-conscious people as a replacement for sugar in the diet and for cooking. It consists mostly of water, fructose, and glucose, a few vitamins and minerals, little or no protein or fat, and only a very small amount of sucrose. Even though the sucrose content is low, and it's considerably less cariogenic than pure sucrose, it does contain other sugars and is sticky, so you should still rinse and brush after eating it.

- ☐ **The rest** All the simple sugars—and there are many, such as maltose, galactose, glucose, and lactose—must be considered cariogenic, if less so than sucrose. The main reasons they're not major contributors to decay are that decay-causing germs don't like them as much as sucrose and almost no one consumes them in the quantities white sugar is consumed.

The bottom line is that if you're serious about eliminating dental disease from your life, you're going to have to read food labels for more than just preservatives and additives. You may even have to carry magnifying glasses around with you to read the super small print (ever notice that the least desirable ingredients are in the tiniest print?). No one is perfect, and there aren't many people who have sucrose-free diets. So do the best you can, and make sure that if you eat anything that contains sugar, any kind of sugar, you rinse your mouth immediately afterward, chew some sugarless gum, and brush as soon as possible.

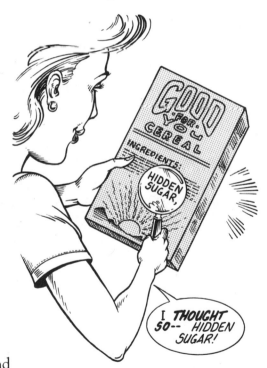

TIPS FOR PARENTS

Very few parents have been able to keep their kids away from sugar. It seems to be found in everything, kids literally become addicted to it, and parents feel they're fighting a hopeless battle. But hold on, there are strategies you can use that work. The three best ways to counteract their sugar addictions, if you can't withdraw them from it, are:

1. Get their dental awareness and hygiene trip together as soon as possible. At least then they'll have the information and hopefully the desire they'll need to minimize, or eliminate, the effects of sugar on their dental health.

2. Introduce them to the principles of sound nutrition.

3. Get them to switch candies. (Granted, this is a compromise solution, but although they'll still be eating sugar, it will be less harmful to their teeth.) Sugar is most harmful to the teeth when it's continually available for the germs to feed on. This means that those candies that remain in the mouth the longest are the worst offenders—the hard sucking candies and the sticky stuff, like caramel and taffy, that are not only sucked on but chewed and that tend to adhere to the teeth. The least harmful to the teeth are the kinds of candy that are quickly disposed of, the ones that go in and down quickly. These don't continually feed the germs like the hard candies, which stay in the mouth a much longer period of time. Explain the difference to your children and get them to switch over. And remind them that they should brush and rinse, or at least chew sugarless gum, as soon as they can after eating any candy.

SOME THINGS TO THINK ABOUT

- ☐ Starches, fats, and protein don't cause decay.
- ☐ Although a sucrose-free diet drastically reduces decay, it does not prevent gum disease. So don't think you can escape oral hygiene because you're sugar free.
- ☐ Sugar eaten with meals is not as cariogenic as sugar eaten between meals. When protein, fats, and starches are included with sucrose the acid created by the sugar-eating germs is, in effect, diluted and is therefore less harmful.

□ Sugar substitutes, such as sorbitol, xylitol, aspartame, saccharin, while not cariogenic, haven't yet been given a clean bill of health when it comes to their long-term effects on the rest of the body. So far, sorbitol and xylitol seem to be the best.

□ No matter how it's sliced and diced, sucrose is the real villain when it comes to decay. You can drastically reduce decay just by eliminating sucrose from your diet. But couple that with a healthy diet and a good hygiene program and you can completely eliminate it.

I know it's not easy to kick any long-term habit, especially diet, but if you do, your efforts will be rewarded a hundred times over. Keep in mind that your teeth and gums are not separate from the rest of your body. If you eat foods that are harmful to your body, they'll be harmful to your teeth and gums. And vice versa—what's harmful to your teeth and gums is not going to be good for the rest of you either. So do the best you can, every little bit helps, and know that you're making a difference.

SUGGESTED READING

Earl Mindell. *The Vitamin Bible*. New York, N.Y.: Warner Books, 1985.

Weston A. Price, D.D.S. *Nutrition and Physical Degeneration*. Order from Nutrition Foundation, Inc., 2901 Wilshire Blvd., Suite 345, Santa Monica, Calif. 90403.

Linda G. Rector-Page, N.D., Ph.D. *Healthy Healing*. Healthy Healing Publications, 1992.

Melvyn R. Werbach, M.D. *Nutritional Influences on Illness*. New Canaan, Conn.: Keats Publishing, 1987.

Dr. Bruce West. *Health Alert Newsletter*. This is an exceptional natural fitness publication. To order it, call 800-231-8063.

Dr. John Yiamouyiannis. *High Performance Health*. Call 614-548-5340 to order.

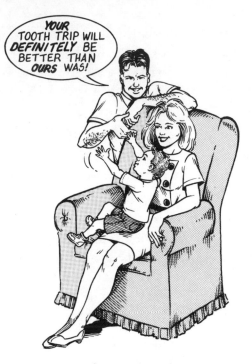

Chapter 17

Parent and Child

When it comes to prevention, you have the opportunity to exercise much more control and influence over the health of your child's mouth than the hygienist or dentist ever can. If you've given up your parental responsibility to the dentist or hygienist, it's now time to take it back. Let the dentist do the repair, and let the hygienist give the preventive support. But you need to do the teaching, set the example, and provide the motivation. Remember, they only see your child a few times a year, but you see her every day. (Before I go further I want to explain that I will be referring to the child as "she." No offense to the male child, but I hope this will somewhat offset the overuse of "he" in our conventional usage.)

This chapter deals with your child's dental trip from preconception through about the age of fifteen, or until she can read *Tooth Fitness*. It also discusses the role the pediatric dentist plays and how to ease your child into good oral hygiene habits.

THE STAGES OF TOOTH DEVELOPMENT

The charts on pages 272–73 show the average ages for the formation and eruption of the baby and permanent teeth (another proof that a few good drawings are worth about 800,000 words). Remember that the ages given on the charts represent the *average*— many children's teeth come in up to a year earlier or later. So don't be concerned if your child's teeth are a little early or late.

The Fetus

The development of the mouth begins when the fetus is about three weeks old, perhaps before you even know you're pregnant (all the more reason to take care of your diet and health all the time— life is full of surprises). The first signs of the baby (*deciduous*) teeth occur at about six weeks. Between the fourth and eighth months the enamel crowns of most of the baby teeth are starting to form, even though the teeth usually don't erupt until months after the baby is born. In fact, shortly before or by the time of birth, even the beginnings of the permanent teeth have been formed.

From Birth to Age Two and a Half

At birth the developing teeth are normally still embedded in the jaws. Generally between four and eight months the front teeth start to erupt. (*Eruption* is when the tooth first starts peeking through the gums.) This is the beginning of the infamous teething stage. By the age of twelve to fifteen months, all the crowns of the baby teeth are formed, although most of them are still hidden in the jaws. The baby teeth continue to erupt until the child is about two and a half, at which time all of them are normally in place. The majority of children end up with twenty baby teeth.

All the while the baby teeth are erupting, the permanent teeth are continuing to develop in the jaw.

From Ages Two and a Half to Six

During this period the permanent teeth continue to grow inside the jaw. The eruption of the first permanent tooth, the six-year molar, occurs between the ages of five and six. These molars come in behind the last baby teeth, which begin to fall out at around six years of age.

STAGES OF TOOTH DEVELOPMENT

PRENATAL
Baby Teeth

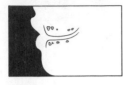 4 months in utero

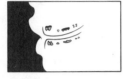 6 months in utero

INFANCY

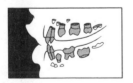 Birth

4 – 8 months

8 – 12 months

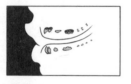 12 – 15 months

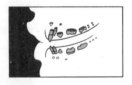 15 – 21 months

EARLY CHILDHOOD

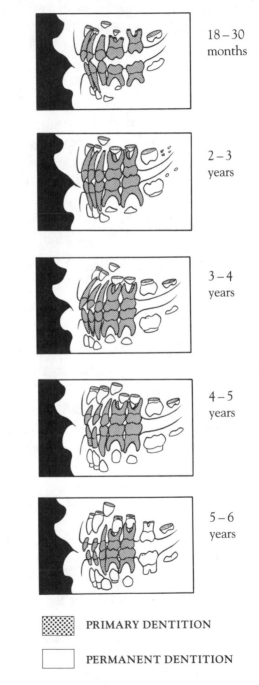

18 – 30 months

2 – 3 years

3 – 4 years

4 – 5 years

5 – 6 years

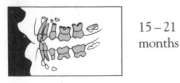

▨ **PRIMARY DENTITION**

☐ **PERMANENT DENTITION**

LATE CHILDHOOD
Mixed Dentition

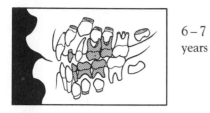

6 – 7
years

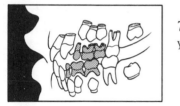

7 – 8
years

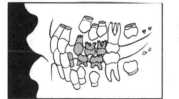

8 – 9
years

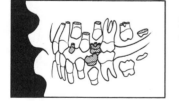

9 – 10
years

ADOLESCENCE
AND ADULTHOOD
Permanent Dentition

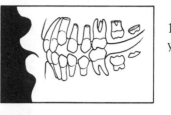

10 – 11
years

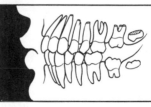

11 – 12
years

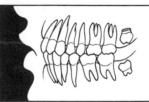

14 – 15
years

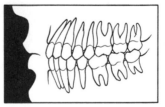

21 years

After Age Six

By fourteen the first twenty-eight permanent teeth usually have erupted. The remaining four wisdom teeth prove not to be as smart as their name implies because it takes them until about age seventeen to make their appearance.

PRECONCEPTION, PREGNANCY, AND NURSING

As a mother you must realize that whatever your baby needs must come from you. While you are your baby's sole source of nutrition, the food you eat is the same food your baby will assimilate. The healthier you are before conception, during pregnancy, and while nursing, the healthier your baby and her teeth will be. Your baby will be receiving the nutrients you assimilated and stored months and even years prior to pregnancy. So, if the food you ingested prior to conception is harmful to you, it'll also be harmful to her—during pregnancy and into the nursing period. If you're planning on a new addition, remember to think ahead.

The development of your baby's mouth begins when the fetus is only three weeks. What this means is that the parts of your child's teeth that will be exposed to the elements outside the womb, and that will have to serve your child for as long as nine to ten years, are forming while the baby is still inside of you and still being fed by you. Your baby's entire prenatal development will be affected by the food you eat. If she can't get the necessary nutrients from you she will simply not be able get it anywhere else. She can't call you on the mobile phone, or jump out and walk to the local health food store. And if she can't get what she needs, the development of her entire oral-facial structure, including her teeth, will be detrimentally affected.

The best way to make sure your baby gets what she needs to develop healthily is to make sure *you* get what *you* need. Empty calories, like white sugar and alcohol, are just that, empty. They do nothing to form healthy bone, teeth, and gums. Eat a healthful diet, make sure you get enough quality protein, and take your vitamins and minerals (especially vitamins A, C, and D and the minerals calcium and phosphorous). Pregnancy places a serious stress on your body and can make your existing gum disease worse, so make sure you're free of all dental disease and have had your teeth repaired.

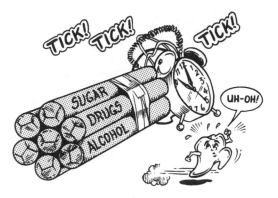

There are other dangers, besides poor nutrition, that can affect your baby's health and development. I'm speaking of drugs, legal ones and illegal ones, all shapes, colors, and doses. Pregnancy is the time not only to watch your food but to pay attention to other substances you may have gotten used to putting into your body. During her first three months in the womb your baby is more sensitive to her environment than she'll ever be during the rest of her life. The development that takes place at this time can't be undone—she only gets one shot at it. So please avoid all drugs, both prescription (unless of course it's a life-threatening situation) and nonprescription, including alcohol, tobacco, and sugar. The harm they can cause your baby now and in the future makes them a time bomb waiting to explode. The gift of prevention begins long before your baby gets her teeth.

If you're not sure about what may or may not be harmful, check in with your common sense, and if that doesn't provide you with the answer, ask your pediatrician. You should also carefully read the nutrition chapter (Chapter 16) and check out the books I recommend there.

BIRTH TO AGE TWO AND A HALF

This is the period when most of the baby teeth erupt. You can check the charts for the average eruption ages. But remember, the eruption ages given are only averages; so don't pay any attention to the old wives' tales that suggest a child is a slow developer or less intelligent if her teeth come in a little later. There's absolutely no evidence to prove that time of tooth eruption is connected to intelligence. But if the eruption dates vary any more than twelve months, and you're concerned, you should consult a pediatric dentist. As the charts show, your baby's first teeth can erupt as early as four months. Occasionally a baby is born with some teeth already in, or they may erupt shortly after birth, but other than the hardship on you during nursing, this is nothing to be concerned about.

Teething Time

Many children have a hard time when it comes to tooth eruption, or *teething*, and some have a very, very hard time of it. Teething can be so traumatic and painful to your baby that you may think there's something wrong, especially if you're a first-time mom. But teething is a normal part of tooth development and growth.

If your baby is irritable, has a slight fever, has congestion, and cries excessively for no apparent reason, you should realize that those symptoms could very well be caused by erupting teeth. If there's no evidence of teething, then look for other causes and check with your pediatrician. Sometimes teething may coincide with an illness, like a cold, and the two problems will serve to magnify each other.

When the chart or your visual examination indicates that eruption is near, or actually taking place, surround the baby with teething toys. Teething toys are thought to help accelerate eruption, massage the gums, and in general help relieve the discomfort. Babies are instinctively wise in this regard, and if they need something and it's within their reach they'll use it. So make sure these gadgets are within your baby's reach during this period—or she'll find something else to do the job. There are many kinds of teething toys on the market. They come in all sizes and shapes and can be found in drugstores, toy stores, or baby stores. The toy ought to be small enough to get far enough into the mouth to be effective, but with a large handle so that she can hold it but not swallow it.

If you have any questions about teething, check with your baby's dentist. He may suggest a specific toy, such as the soft plastic kind that has water inside. This can be placed in your freezer compartment and frozen. Cold not only provides the desired numbing

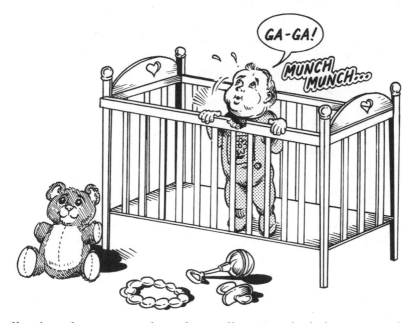

effect but also acts to reduce the swelling. Let the baby use it on her own, if she will. But if the coldness bothers her fingers and she refuses, or if she's just too upset and distracted with pain, you use it for her. Move it lightly around the affected area with a gentle massage action. It will act both as an anesthetic and a massager. If she wants to chew on it, let her. Do this for a little while; then wait ten minutes, and repeat as needed. Don't keep it on the gum area for more than a minute at a time.

If a tooth has broken through and the area around it is red and swollen, you can mix about one ounce of 3 percent hydrogen peroxide with one ounce of warm water, stir well, and apply this solution with a cotton swab. There are also teething solutions available at your drug store, from your pediatrician, and from the children's dentist that are specifically formulated to reduce the physical discomforts of teething. However, I recommend you try these only as a last resort because they may contain chemicals, mostly benzocaine. Hylands, a maker of homeopathic remedies, has a teething formula that is natural and harmless, and I've heard from many mothers that it's effective.

Once all the baby teeth have erupted, you and your child will be free from the trauma of teething. The first permanent tooth won't erupt until about the age of six. This is great news for both of you, so enjoy the break while you can. When the permanent teeth start arriving you'll both have to go through it again, although it's normally less traumatic the second time around. If a teething problem arises with the permanent teeth, use the same procedures you used with the baby teeth.

Breast and Bottle Feeding

Scientists have proven what our ancestors knew for millions of years, that there's no food as nutritionally complete as a healthy mother's milk. It supplies everything your baby needs to grow. Think about that . . . *no other food can make that claim*. And, if you've taken care of your diet, it contains no additives, preservatives, or artificial flavors. It's also free.

There's evidence that breast-fed babies have jaws and teeth that are better and more completely developed than formula-fed babies. If you can't breast-feed, for whatever reason, talk to your pediatrician or health food store nutritional consultant about infant vitamin supplements.

Potential Problems with the Breast and the Bottle

Once all the baby teeth are in place, the child's pre-teeth swallowing pattern will change to an adult swallowing pattern as the tongue adapts to the shape of the new teeth. This adult pattern comes naturally to the child as soon as all her baby teeth come in— if she doesn't have a bottle to suck on all the time. But if the child is allowed more than occasional contact with the bottle or the breast after her teeth have arrived, the suckling action puts unnatural pressure on the new teeth. The tongue thrusts forward and pushes against the front teeth, and consequently she could end up with buck teeth. These pressures can also lead to other jaw and teeth deformities.

A child's bones are very soft and pliable and can also become deformed very easily. A simple act, such as continuously sleeping with her hands under her face, on the bottle, or on a toy, could cause problems. So keep an eye on your child's sleeping habits. If you notice that she sleeps in the same position most of the time, gently rearrange her hands or remove any object she's sleeping on. It's important to catch these potentially harmful patterns early, before they become harder-to-break habits later.

Always check the ingredients of any formula or baby food you feed your baby. If it contains sugar, avoid it like the plague. There's no sense beginning her sugar addiction any sooner than you're forced to. You can find plenty of healthy formulas and baby foods without sugar. Check your local health food store; they carry some nutritious and natural baby formulas.

If you use the bottle, *never*, and I mean *never*, leave a bottle of milk or juice in your baby's crib at night. As you well know, she'll let you know when she's hungry, but when she finishes drinking, be sure to take the bottle away. You may get a little less sleep waiting for her to finish, but her teeth will be a lot healthier.

Why? Because if your baby goes to sleep with the bottle in her mouth the strong acids found in the milk or juice will remain in contact with the teeth all night. These acids can quickly etch away the thin enamel of the baby teeth. It's like letting her suck on candy all night. You wouldn't let her do that, would you? If you feel you must leave a bottle in the crib at night, fill it with water. Also, it's a good idea to give your baby a bottle with water in it after feeding her milk or juice during waking hours. It's an excellent way to rinse her mouth of the acidic and sugary milk or juice.

Thumb Sucking and Pacifiers

Thumb sucking is a normal habit for an infant. By the age of two or so, the baby usually stops on her own. But if your baby continues to suck her thumb after the baby teeth have erupted, it could lead to serious bite problems. To discourage this habit will take patience and diligence on your part, and you should begin as soon as her baby teeth have arrived. If you don't, the result will be unsightly teeth and possibly costly orthodontics later on.

Many dentists will tell you not to give your child a pacifier at any time because sucking on it could develop into a hard-to-break habit. If she's allowed to continue using a pacifier after the baby teeth have come in, it could cause the same problems as thumb sucking does.

If either of these habits is a problem, and you can't seem to resolve it on your own, tell your dentist. He can help you and your child deal with it in a number of ways, such as providing counseling and/or devices that are designed to discourage the habit.

Examining Your Baby's Teeth

The enamel of baby teeth is usually not as thick or hard as the enamel of permanent teeth (the baby teeth only have to stay around for ten years or so), and decay can move so fast that periodic examinations by you and the pediatric dentist are a must. But especially by you. I've always thought of baby teeth as practice teeth— meaning you get a chance to get your child's hygiene trip together before her permanent teeth arrive. But that doesn't mean you can neglect the baby teeth.

You can do your part by keeping your eye on your child's teeth between dental visits. It's a good idea to write down the dates you examine her and what you find. Once a month is a good schedule to start with. You'll find a page called "Baby's Tooth Diary" in the Appendix that you can use for this purpose. If you do this you'll be able to monitor her and assess how well the two of you are doing, and if something isn't normal you can alert the dentist. This "diary" can also be very valuable to the pediatric dentist or orthodontist when it comes to evaluating her dental history. I think your child will also appreciate being able to look back on these notes when she grows up.

AGES TWO AND A HALF TO SIX

This is a critical period. You'll need to pay close attention to see if your child's teeth are coming in properly. Use the charts to follow the eruption process. Normally, the baby teeth erupt by two and a half, but sometimes the process continues to age four. If the teeth come in crowded, or aren't properly aligned, or if there are signs of decay, you should make an appointment to see the dentist. Once you've gotten her on a regular checkup program and have had the teeth repaired, the most important thing you can do during this period is to make sure you get her involved with oral hygiene. I talk about how to do that later in the chapter.

AGE SIX TO *TOOTH FITNESS*

The Eruption of the Permanent Teeth

At, or around, the age of six, two things happen to a child's mouth:

1. The first four permanent molars erupt. This may happen easily, or it may be difficult and painful. The tops of the molars are very broad and can create havoc with the gums when breaking through the skin.

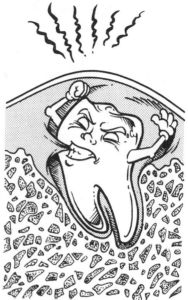

As the tooth erupts, it slowly pushes through the gum tissue, often leaving a flap of tissue over-hanging the tooth. If food gets jammed under this flap, the irrita-tion and the toxins released by the germs eating the impacted food may cause the gums to become sore, swollen, and painful. This could turn into a gum infection, or even an abscess, either of which could cause more swelling, more pain, and possibly even a fever. So at the first sign of irritation, fol-low the directions for problem wisdom teeth in the dental emer-gency chapter (page 213). If home treatment doesn't help, call and make an appointment with her dentist. If she's in a lot of pain and tolerates aspirin, you can give her the recommended dose of chil-dren's aspirin, or whatever other pain reliever your doctor may rec-ommend. If need be, the dentist can easily cut and clean the area, and eruption will proceed normally.

2. She starts to lose her baby teeth (review the eruption chart for the dates). In a sense, the permanent teeth push the baby teeth out. Under pressure from the permanent teeth the roots of the baby teeth dissolve. Since the teeth are no longer firmly anchored in the jaw, they loosen more and more until they fall out. This is why, when the baby teeth fall out normally, there are no roots to be seen. So you can let the baby teeth fall out of their own accord (they've

been falling out on their own for millions of years). Or, if a tooth seems to be taking an inordinate amount of time, the child can't stand it hanging around anymore, and the permanent tooth is scheduled for arrival, you can have the pediatric dentist take it out.

Checking for Proper Alignment

The proper positioning and alignment of the baby teeth is the key to the proper eruption of the four six-year molars, which can erupt as early as five. If the six-year molars (which, in case you forgot, are permanent teeth) come in correctly, the chances are excellent (if the jaws are big enough) that the rest of the permanent teeth will do the same.

The main reasons permanent teeth don't erupt properly have to do with crowded or misaligned baby teeth, the premature loss of baby teeth, and the loss of tooth structure because of untreated decay at the contact points. When the spacing of the baby teeth is not normal and they move too close together, the six-year molars, which come in directly behind the last baby teeth, will be positioned too far forward. This means there will be less space in the jaw for the permanent teeth that will erupt in front of the six-year molars. The result is crowding of the permanent teeth.

You'll be able to see obvious crowding problems and if there is advanced decay, but it'll take a dentist's evaluation to determine the extent of the problem and the most advisable way to treat it. If you haven't taken your child to the pediatric dentist yet, you should do so before the six-year molars erupt, when she's five, especially if her baby teeth are already crowded. This could save you from costly orthodontic problems later on.

If her six-year molars erupt properly and the dentist gives her a clean bill of health, the rest of her permanent teeth should come in without any problem (teething being a possible exception). Keep up with your home checkups, but unless you see something that isn't normal, from here on out your biggest concern will be her oral hygiene.

THE PEDIATRIC DENTIST (PEDODONTIST)

I discuss the role of the pediatric dentist here because he deals strictly with children, whereas the orthodontist, who is discussed along with the other dental specialists in Chapter 12, deals with big people too. The pediatric dentist is a dentist who has chosen to undergo additional schooling to allow him to specialize in children's dentistry. Pediatric dentists are usually listed in the phone book under Dentists, subheading Pediatrics, or, as they were previously known, Pedodontists.

The pediatric dentist is valuable even if your child never has a dental problem. He can, through periodic checkups, confirm your home evaluations and work with you to establish a preventive program for her. If she has *any* dental problems the pediatric dentist is always the one to call first. Use the guidelines in Chapter 6, "Finding a Dentist and a Dental Hygienist," to find one.

If you can't find a pediatric dentist in your town, don't hesitate to take your child to a general dentist, either your own personal dentist or a different one. Yours may be great for you, but he might not like to work on children. If he isn't the one for her, please don't force him on your child, or vice versa, just because it's convenient or you don't want to offend him. If you must take her to a general dentist, I suggest you ask him if he sees many children and if he has any problem working with kids. Be out front about this, because he may not offer you that information. You'll would be doing yourself, the dentist, and especially your child a favor if you find out how he feels before the appointments begin.

I don't mean to suggest that a general dentist isn't capable of treating many of your child's dental problems; nor am I saying that all pediatric dentists get along perfectly with every child. What I am saying is that the possibility of problems arising, especially if the child is between the ages of one and ten, is greater if you take your child to just any general dentist. I say this because the child still has most of her baby teeth, and in most cases the pediatric dentist simply has more experience in this area. Also his office is designed with children in mind, is usually more acceptable to kids, and the child feels more comfortable among her peers. She sees that other children are there—so why not her? I'd take my children to a pediatric dentist, and that's the best recommendation I could give.

The Child/Dentist Relationship

When you take your child to the dentist, pay extremely close attention to the relationship that develops between them. Listen to what your child has to say about it, and if you think there's a problem discuss it openly with the dentist. Never, *ever*, force a bad dental experience upon her.

If you force the child on the dentist, or vice versa, not only may she become afraid of that dentist and lose confidence in him, but she could transfer those feelings to her future dentists. If the experience is bad enough and leads her to believe that all dentists are the same, it could keep her from going to the dentist at all after she leaves home and is on her own. And that could be a long-term disaster when it comes to her oral health. It could also be an experience the child might never forgive you for. If a satisfactory solution can't be reached—satisfactory to all three of you—it would be better to try a new dentist. Don't blame; simply make a change.

When to Take Her and Why

Many pediatric dentists recommend a first appointment when the child is between twelve and eighteen months old (some even suggest six months), and certainly no later than two and a half (when all her baby teeth have erupted). If you take her at twelve months the chances are very good that this will be a problem-free visit and a positive experience for her.

Also, if she has problems in any of the categories below, or if you see anything else that doesn't seem normal, take her to the pediatric dentist as soon as you can get an appointment:

- ☐ Her teeth show signs of decay. Some children develop decay shortly after a tooth erupts, and about 50 percent of all two-year-olds have at least one cavity.
- ☐ She's had a serious fall or blow to the head. Take her whether you think there's a problem or not.
- ☐ Her diet has contained an excessive amount of sugar.
- ☐ She has genetic problems affecting the teeth or jaws (e.g., her lower jaw seems to protrude too far forward or is recessed).
- ☐ Her baby teeth have not erupted properly or are crowded.

What Does the Pediatric Dentist Do?

Unless it's an emergency, the first appointment with the dentist will consist of a "getting to know each other" type of examination. It's important that this visit be a happy one, not scary or painful. What happens at the first-ever visit could determine the pattern of all your child's future dental visits. Depending on her age, she may already have heard negative stories about going to the dentist. There are enough such stories floating around; a few may be true, but most aren't. So don't feed her imagination with negative thoughts about the dentist, even if you yourself have had a bad experience. The pediatric dentist is well aware that an uneventful first visit is the perfect time to make a bond with the child in a positive way. And if you as a parent can be a support, be a pal, and make it fun—it could help her formulate a positive attitude toward dentists that could last her a lifetime.

If the dentist doesn't want you in the room, heed his wish. He's had lots of experience with all kinds of kids, so give him a chance to do what he does best. Often children try to use their parents as a crutch, show off, or try to pit you against the dentist. Be understanding and caring, but stand firm.

If you take your child to the dentist before she has any problems, he'll examine her mouth, take X rays (depending on her age and what he sees), possibly give her a fluoride treatment (I discuss fluoride in Chapter 18) and a cleaning. He'll also give her some hygiene guidance (again depending on her age). And that will be it.

If there's a problem, the dentist will have her back and present you with a treatment plan and schedule. If there's decay, she'll have to have fillings or stainless steel crowns placed, depending on the extent of it. If the decay involves the nerve and the dentist feels the tooth must be saved to maintain proper spacing, he may have to do what is called a *pulpotomy* (removal of the upper portion of the nerve), or a *pulpectomy* (removal of the entire nerve, commonly called a *root canal*). In some cases a tooth, or teeth, may have to be extracted and a *space maintainer* made to keep the rest of the teeth from moving. Your dentist will also evaluate her for possible orthodontic work and either do it himself or refer her to an orthodontist.

Fully utilize the pediatric dentist and the hygienist. Keep in mind that he and his staff won't be afraid to answer any questions you may have, so don't be afraid to ask. Never be satisfied with an answer you don't understand. You are paying for your right to know. Not just for you, but for your child too.

TEACHING YOUR CHILD
THE TECHNIQUES OF HOME CARE

Because habits are easier to make than to break, it's a lifetime gift to your child to help her establish good dental habits right away. There are various ways to introduce your child to brushing techniques and other home care procedures. I'll offer you some effective methods, but be sure to also ask your pediatric dentist and the hygienist for their input and guidance. They'll be able to tell you which areas of your child's mouth are being well cared for and which may need more attention. It's also beneficial to the child to be told how well she's doing by people other than yourself, like the dentist and hygienist. Kids, big ones and small ones, like positive feedback, and positive feedback is super important in any learning process. Use the dentist as you would a guide in a foreign country, and never turn down his help.

The Early Years

Until your child is old enough to take care of her own hygiene you'll have to it for her. Lay your baby on your lap and gently clean her teeth with a 2-by-2-inch gauze pad or a clean cloth. This is a good way to introduce her to the process of teeth cleaning. As she gets older replace the gauze with a small, soft child's brush, but be gentle and make it a loving adventure.

The first, and most effective, way to begin teaching your child home care is to expose her to the philosophy of prevention at an early age, and to do it as often as possible. These are the years when many habits are easily and quickly formed, so it's a critical stage of life. And since it's just as easy to follow in the footsteps of a good habit as it is a bad one, now is the perfect opportunity to get a good dental one going for her.

As soon as she can toddle, take her with you whenever you brush. Do this even before you let her play with brushing her own teeth; it will help prepare her for that event. The best time to do this is after every meal (but of course you knew that, didn't you?), especially when your child eats with you. You don't have to wake her up and drag her to the bathroom; you want this to be a positive experience. Make a big deal out of it—"We get to brush now!"—not we "have" to brush now. Talk to her and explain what you're doing, even if she doesn't fully understand yet. Gargle and make funny sounds; let her hold the brush. When you rinse, see if you can get her to rinse too. Whatever you do, try to make it fun. It's one of those positive experiences in which by helping yourself you also help someone you love.

Next, introduce her to brushing. Get the smallest brush you can find, with the softest bristles. The best guideline to follow is the smaller the child the smaller the brush. The soft brushes are gentler on the delicate tissues of your child's mouth. If you can find a brush with a soft rubber handle you can give it to your child before all her teeth come in and perhaps she'll take to it as a teething toy. Try your pediatric dentist, or look for it in the drugstore. After she's watched you do your tooth workout for a few weeks, and you think she's ready, introduce her to the brush. The infant's and child's brushes that I like the best are made by Butler.

Don't use any toothpaste at first, not until she can be taught how to rinse and spit without swallowing. Just wet the brush and tell her you're going to show her how to brush like Mommy (or Daddy). There's no set way to do this. *Just be patient and don't force it.* Watch her closely. Adjust the handle and her movements when necessary so that the brush, not the handle, is on the teeth and going in the right direction. Don't worry too much about the movement, but gently make the corrections so her motion is the same as yours. Have her brush with you sometimes while you're looking at each other and, at other times, while you're both looking in the mirror. As you know, most kids tend to get bored easily, so vary it, approach it from all angles. As the little one's coordination improves so will her technique. It really won't take that long before she'll get it down.

When she can handle it, you can add toothpaste. She'll most likely demand it because you're using it. I strongly suggest that you get a natural toothpaste, made by a manufacturer who isn't afraid to list the ingredients on the label. (I recommend Tom's of Maine.) Most commercial toothpastes have ingredients in them that, while they may or may not be all right for use in the mouth, are definitely not meant to be swallowed—especially by a child. She won't know this though, especially if it tastes good. Children between the ages of two and six swallow about a third of the toothpaste they put into their mouths. Those between the ages of seven to sixteen swallow about 20 percent of it. Because most toothpastes, especially the ones targeting children, contain fluoride, it's important to keep your child from swallowing them. This is even more critical if she's already getting fluoride in her drinking water, rinses, and fluoride treatments. Remember, children are much more susceptible to chemicals than adults. There's enough fluoride in a medium tube of toothpaste to make a child seriously ill, if she should eat all of it; it could even be fatal. So treat fluoridated toothpaste as a medicine, and never leave it within your child's reach.

You may have to try different flavors before you find one that your child likes. This may seem like a frivolous concern, but it isn't really. A toothpaste that tastes bad could turn her off to brushing altogether. Also, you don't need to use very much paste—just a pea-sized dab will do her. If the toothpaste contains fluoride use no more than a third of a pea-sized dab.

Aim to brush with her after every meal. Or have her brush her teeth in the morning and you brush them for her before bedtime. That way she still gets to practice and you get to make sure she doesn't miss any spots.

As far as flossing goes, you yourself will have to get the technique down pat before you can teach it. (See Chapter 5.) Once you do, you can introduce it to your child. Start with the front teeth because they're the easiest. This will give her confidence. Coordination is the key here, more than age. Try it when she's about six and see how she does. Once she gets the front teeth down, move on to the back teeth. Don't force it or make it a chore. If she can't grasp it, it isn't because she doesn't want to but because she doesn't yet have the dexterity to do it. Let it go for a while and reintroduce it later. If you have patience, she'll master it in time.

If you have more than one child, especially if you have three or more, it may be difficult for you to find the time to stay on top of their oral hygiene program. One way to make it easier on yourself and to get your children more involved is to enlist the help of your oldest child as your hygiene assistant. Tell her you'll be teaching her everything she needs to know about preventing dental disease and you want her to help teach the other kids. She'll get more involved with her own mouth, and she'll also feel valuable and important.

You can monitor the process by sitting in while she's teaching the younger kids and then periodically checking their brushing skills and examining their mouths after they've brushed. Do this daily at first, and if it's successful you can taper off to every few days. The age at which the oldest child will be able to do this will vary, but you can start as soon as she understands what role you want her to play and is able to master the skills herself. It may take a while, but it'll be well worth the time you initially spend teaching her. You'll be pleasantly surprised at the results and by how much time it'll save you later on. Peer pressure can be positive.

Another valuable teaching tool is disclosing tablets. (I speak about them on page 113 in Chapter 4.) Disclosing tablets colorfully stain plaque and food debris and is a wonderful way to show your child where she's done a good job and where she hasn't. Use them once a week until you're sure she's gotten her brushing and flossing skills down. You can get them from your dentist or drugstore.

As Your Child Grows

Up until the time your child goes to school you'll be the major influence on her dental life, and it's during these early years that you'll have the best opportunity to counteract the harmful pressures she'll have to face as she grows older. By the time your child starts school she should be so familiar with the prevention techniques and helpful little tricks you've taught her that practicing oral hygiene will be as natural as breathing air. Have her read *Tooth Fitness* as soon as she's able to. She won't understand everything at first, but you can answer her questions.

Remember to keep up with regular home and office checkups, and always chart and record everything you see that may not be normal. By doing this and getting feedback from your dentist as to where she needs to spend more time brushing, you'll be able to make an accurate evaluation of your child's brushing and home care habits. In this way you'll be able to continue to monitor and direct her preventive program until she has it down cold.

The ages between six and eighteen could be the most difficult ages she'll go through, dentally speaking. What with peer pressure, media advertising promoting junk food and the "sugar experience," and the seeming inability of kids and teens to make enough time for their oral health, her teeth will literally be at war with her environment. You must do your best to help her through this traumatic period. Obviously you can't brush her teeth for her or follow her around and take her candy away from her, but you can, and must, make sure she is armed with knowledge.

Using threats and scare tactics isn't the best way to motivate teenagers. The most effective way I've found to reach them is to appeal to their sense of vanity. Have your dentist or hygienist show your teenager pictures of severe decay and gum disease so she can actually see what can result if she doesn't take care of her mouth. Then simply ask her if she would date someone whose mouth was in such a condition. When she says no, ask her if she thinks someone would want to date her if her mouth looked like that. Also, ask her opinion of her peers who have rotting teeth, unsightly gums, and bad breath. This approach works wonders. You could also have her read Chapter 15, "Dentures and Implants."

Remember, your responsibility as a parent isn't to *make* her do what she should, but to give her the information she'll need to make her *want* to do what she should do. Knowledge will set you both free.

A FEW MORE IMPORTANT THINGS

Sealants

If your child is decay-prone, your dentist may suggest applying a sealant to the occlusal surfaces of the back teeth. This is an inexpensive procedure that creates a barrier against food, bacteria, and plaque—very effective at preventing decay in these highly susceptible areas. A sealant is a thin layer of composite material that is literally painted on the teeth. First the dentist will clean the grooves of plaque and food debris; then he'll fill in the grooves and defects with the sealant. Sealants should be done as soon as possible after the baby and permanent teeth erupt. They will periodically have to be redone, though some will last as long as three to five years. If you're against fluoride or it isn't available, sealants are a must. I highly recommend them.

Cosmetic Treatment

Cosmetic dentistry is available for children, and most pediatric dentists are experienced with it. See Chapter 13 for a full discussion.

Mouth-Guards

After decay and gum disease, accidental injury to the teeth is the most commonly seen dental problem for those under eighteen. Most injuries are the result of contact sports, such as football, basketball, baseball, hockey, and soccer; but many result from bike riding, skiing, skate boarding, and roller blading, or from general roughhousing. These injuries often could have been prevented by mouth-guards. Prefabricated mouth-guards can be purchased at sporting goods stores, but the best ones are custom-made at the dental office.

Study Models

Study models are inexpensive plaster models of the teeth. I recommend you ask the dentist to make a set (uppers and lowers) for your child after her permanent teeth have come in. If she ever has an accident and loses one or more teeth the dentist will be able to use the model as a guide to accurately replace them. You should have your own set made, for the same reason. Even if the dentist has a set, you should keep one set at home.

Lost Teeth

If a permanent tooth is knocked out intact, there's a good chance it can be replanted if you can get your child and the tooth to the dentist within thirty minutes to an hour. The chance of success decreases with time. You probably won't be with her at the time of the accident, so here's what she should know. Tell her to pick up the tooth by the crown, not the root. Then gently rinse it and place it in a cloth moistened with water or milk. Next she should call the dentist. She should tell the receptionist it's an emergency and get there ASAP. She should always carry the name and phone number of her dentist with her.

Premedication and General Anesthesia

Some children, no matter what you or the dentist do to try to prevent it, will be overly fearful at the dental office. Or sometimes a traumatic situation, such an accident, requires especially painful and extensive treatment. If you go to a pediatric dentist, he'll be well prepared for these situations because he's skilled in the art of minimizing the negative aspects of your child's dental experience. When all other means of relieving your child's anxiety have failed, he may want to recommend premedication—the administration of certain drugs, or gas, for the purpose of eliminating pain, anxiety, and fear. He'll suggest this in order to calm her enough so that the necessary work can get done.

Talk it over with the dentist. Sometimes premedication or general anesthesia is not only the right choice but the only one. If anesthesia is indicated the dental work may have to be done at a hospital. Discuss your feelings with the dentist and make sure you know exactly what will be done and what you can expect. And be sure to check with your dentist and doctor about possible allergies or other side effects from the drug being used before you allow it to be administered.

Special Situations

If your child is chronically ill or handicapped, special planning will be required, and the pediatric dentist, working closely with your physician, will be the best person to deal with the situation.

FINANCIAL CONSIDERATIONS

I realize you may not be able to follow all of my advice about treatment. Dentistry certainly isn't inexpensive. But it is necessary, and when it's put off, for any reason, it always ends up costing more in the long run. You should, at the very least, find the money to have your child examined and have any potential problems treated on a temporary basis. I wish I had a magic wand to wave away the money problems, but since I don't I'll offer some suggestions.

Tell your dentist about your financial situation. He may be able to set up a program in which the most serious problems can be treated first and the rest treated as you can afford to pay for them. Or you might be able to set up a workable payment schedule. Many dentists will allow this, especially if they know you're willing to do your part in regard to prevention. Also, look into all of the various governmental assistance programs available. You can also call your local dental association and ask if there's a free clinic. Many caring dentists get together to offer free clinics for those financially unable to pay for their child's dental treatment. Do the best you can, but I

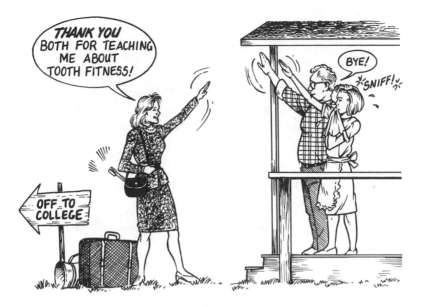

can tell you, with complete certainty, that if your difficulty is money, prevention is answer. *Tooth Fitness* may not be able to repair the damage already done, but it can definitely get you and your child involved in the practice of prevention and free you both from future dental disease.

IN SUMMARY

This chapter isn't about teaching you how to be your child's dentist. What I hope to have gotten across to you is that you're the one mainly responsible for the health of your child's mouth. It's you who'll have the biggest influence on your child's dental education. In order to do your job well, you'll have to know what she'll have to know, and you'll have to be willing to take the time to teach it.

SUGGESTED READING

Arlene Eisenberg. *What to Eat When Expecting.* New York: Workman Publishing, 1986.

James F. Fries, M.D., Robert H. Pantell, M.D., and Donald M. Vickery, M.D. *Taking Care of Your Child.* Reading, Mass.: Addison-Wesley Publishing, 1990. (This is a great book, like the *Tooth Fitness* of parent-child medical care. Every parent should have a copy.)

Leo Galland, M.D. *Superimmunity for Kids.* New York: Copestone Press, 1988.

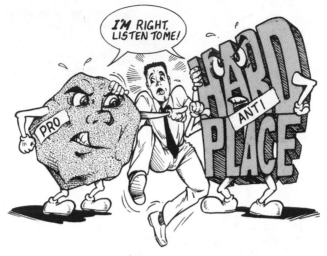

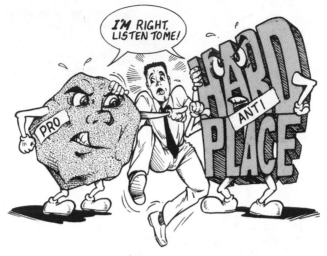
I'M RIGHT, LISTEN TO ME!

PRO

HARD
ANTI
PLACE

Chapter 18

Fluoride and Mercury

If there are any more controversial subjects in the field of dentistry I don't know what they would be. Millions of dollars have been spent and millions of words have been written in an attempt to decide whether or not to fluoridate water and whether or not the use of mercury in dental fillings is harmful. To date, all efforts to resolve these often emotional controversies have failed. If the experts on both sides still can't agree, where does that leave *you*? You're right— about halfway between a rock and a hard place.

My aim here is to untangle the threads of the controversy and clear up your confusion. I believe that with the information in this chapter you'll be able to make informed decisions. The approach I take is a practical one, exploring what will work for you in the real world. But if you happen to be interested in the nitty gritty, scientific details, I'll tell you where to look at the end of the chapter.

FLUORIDE

What It Is and How It Works

No matter how complicated the fluoridation issue can be made out to be, the principles behind it are really quite simple. The purpose of of using fluoride is to reduce or eliminate the tooth's susceptibility to decay. It can do this in two ways, either by actually becoming incorporated into the tooth structure or by topical application to the tooth surface.

How fluoride becomes part of the enamel Enamel is a combination of the elements calcium, phosphorous, oxygen, and hydrogen. Its formula is $Ca_5(PO_4)_3OH$, and it's called *hydroxyapatite*. Before the enamel of a tooth is formed, a matrix, in the shape of the tooth, develops at the site in the jaw where the tooth will form (this matrix is something like the frame of a house). Then the dentin is deposited within the matrix, and the enamel is laid down on top of the dentin to form the crown. The crowns of the teeth always develop before the roots. (The charts on pages 272–73 show when and how long it takes the enamel to form.)

The thickness of the tooth's enamel varies, from .5 mm at the place where the enamel ends on the root surface to 1.5 mm at the cusps, where it gets the most wear. Barring any problems, the process of depositing the enamel continues until all the enamel of the crown has formed.

During this process, if enough fluoride (from food, from natural fluoride in the water, or from fluoridated water) finds its way via the blood to the forming enamel, the fluoride molecule has the opportunity to compete with the *hydroxy radical* (OH) to see which will mate with the phosphate molecule. It so happens that the fluoride molecule has a much stronger attraction to the phosphate molecule than its competitor. When the fluoride succeeds in replacing the hydroxy radical, the enamel formula changes to $Ca_5(PO_4)_3F$ and is called *fluorapatite*. In this way, if fluoride is accessible when the crowns are forming, it becomes part of the enamel.

People generally think the tooth becomes harder when fluoride has been added in this way to the enamel. This isn't the case. It doesn't become harder in the sense that a diamond is harder than glass. What happens is that the tooth, with the addition of fluoride, becomes more resistant to the acid produced by bacteria. It's believed that the addition of fluoride fights decay in three ways: by making the enamel less soluble by the acids that germs produce, by reducing the ability of germs to produce acid, and by reducing the number of germs in plaque that is attached to the enamel.

If, from the moment the enamel begins to form until it's completely formed, there's enough fluoride available, every minute of every day, then all the enamel will contain fluoride. If this ideal situation occurs, fluoride will be found throughout the entire thickness of the enamel, and the enamel will be more resistant to the acid that initiates decay. However, if the intake of fluoride is interrupted during crown formation, the part of the enamel being formed at that particular time won't be protected by fluoride. In fact, even if fluoride is available to the teeth during the entire formation process, some areas (such as the occlusal grooves of the back teeth, pits, and other defects) may not be protected as well because the enamel is very thin and because those areas act as plaque traps (which allow decay-causing acid to concentrate).

In my opinion, fluoridation of the water is an attempt to "vaccinate" the public against tooth decay, somewhat like vaccinating to prevent measles or polio. But although some diseases can be prevented by a simple vaccination or two, protecting the teeth against decay is more complicated. If you wanted maximum protection with fluoride, instead of a few vaccinations you would have to drink about two quarts of water fluoridated at the recommended level—0.7 to 1.2 ppm (1 ppm is equal to one part fluoride in a million parts of water)—every single day, for as long as twelve to fourteen years (the time it takes for the enamel of the baby and permanent teeth to form). The protection you receive is directly related to when you ingest the fluoride, how much is available, and how long it was taken.

Topical fluoride Even if fluoride isn't systemically available to the enamel while it's forming inside the jaw, it can still play a role in preventing decay if it's topically applied to the surfaces of the teeth after they've erupted. Topical fluoride, whether applied directly to the teeth at the dental office or applied through the use of fluoride toothpastes, fluoride mouthwashes, or fluoridated water, helps *remineralize* the surface layers of the enamel or dentin—that is, it helps to replace the minerals that acids have etched from the surface layers of the teeth. This process is a lot like repainting a wall whose paint has worn off. Although other minerals found in the mouth from saliva and foods can contribute to remineralization, fluoride has been shown to be the most effective.

The Controversy

Even the controversy is controversial. The profluoride faction seems content to limit the issue solely to how much fluoride is safe to use in fluoridated water, while the antifluoride faction takes a broader perspective. Those supporting water fluoridation say that at the level of 0.7 to 1.2 ppm, fluoride in the water system isn't harmful to the teeth or the body. Those against fluoridating the water system are divided into three general camps: those who believe that anything more than naturally found trace amounts of fluoride not only is unnecessary but can be toxic, and who are therefore against fluoridation of water as well as against any other artificial fluoride; those who see it as a freedom-of-choice issue; and those who feel it's both.

Both sides strongly support their positions, not only with their own interpretations of the available research material (and accusations that the opposition's research is flawed, skewed, incomplete, misunderstood, etc.) but also with emotion and propaganda. So let's take a look at some of the facts.

Fluoride Facts You Should Know

I know it sounds a little silly, but I think you need a few introductory facts to help understand the facts that will follow.

At the level of 1 ppm of fluoride, which is what most fluoridated water systems use, a quart of water will contain about 1 mg (milligram) of fluoride, or about 1/28,350 of an ounce. This may seem like an almost infinitesimal amount of fluoride (so what's the big fuss about?) until you consider a couple of other factors. One, various health organizations set the optimum daily intake for adults at 1 to 1.2 mg per day and the *maximum safe allowance* at as little as 1.5 to 5 mg per day. And, two, you get fluoride from other sources besides drinking water.

Okay, now let's get to the rest of the facts.

1. Artificially fluoridated drinking water was introduced in the 1940s. Today about 60 percent of the population in the United States (150 million people) have access to fluoridated water. Much research has been done to determine its effectiveness at reducing decay, and although some studies suggest it has little or no value, fluoridated water is generally believed to be anywhere between 20 and 60 percent effective.

2. More than eighty organizations, including the World Health Organization (WHO), the National Institute of Dental Research (NIDR), the American Dental Association (ADA), and the American Cancer Society, state that at the recommended levels fluoridated water is safe.

3. The National Research Council recognizes fluorine as an essential trace element for the body. The tentatively recommended maximum daily amount of fluoride considered safe is based on weight. It ranges from 0.1 to 1 mg for infants, 0.5 to 1.5 mg for children, 1.5 to 2.5 mg for teenagers, and 1.5 to 4 mg for adults. WHO has set the maximum safe daily intake of fluoride for adults at 5 mg. However, not everyone thinks it's necessary to health; the National Academy of Sciences, for instance, says fluoride isn't an essential nutrient.

4. Of the more than one hundred chemical elements (such as oxygen, hydrogen, and carbon), fluorine is the thirteenth most abundant, which means there's a lot of it around. It's found naturally in soil, water, air, plants, and animals.

5. In the United States fluoride found naturally in fresh water ranges from about 1 ppm in the Northeast to over 10 ppm in certain areas of the Southwest. Seawater contains about 1.5 ppm.

6. Most foods (fruits, vegetables, meat, and seafood) contain fluoride. Fruits and vegetables, depending on where they are grown and whether fluoridated water is used to irrigate and process them, can contain more than 0.2 mg per serving, with lettuce and spinach leading the pack. Seafood is high in fluoride, especially shellfish, salmon, sardines, and mackerel.

7. Fluoride is considered more toxic than lead, is fatal in high doses, and has produced toxic side effects in lesser doses. It's been used as a pesticide and as a rodent poison. A single dose of 5 grams (a little less than one-fifth of an ounce) is lethal to an adult human, and 1 gram or less is lethal to a small child. Twenty to 80 mg is considered toxic, and as little as 4 to 8 mg ingested daily while the enamel is forming can cause dental *fluorosis* (discoloration, pitting, and structural damage to enamel; also called *mottling*).

8. Dental fluorosis is increasing. About 30 percent of children show some signs of mottling. The extent of the mottling is deter-

mined by how much excess fluoride finds its way to the enamel, when it's ingested, and for how long it's ingested.

9. Fluoride allergies have been reported to result from as little as the recommended fluoridated water intake of 1.2 mg per day. The symptoms exhibited were fatigue, dizziness, skin rash, joint pain, stomach problems, nausea, and vomiting. They subsided when the fluoridated water intake was stopped. Other studies find no evidence of allergies with recommended doses.

10. Studies have shown that people with existing kidney problems can be affected by drinking water with as little as 2 ppm fluoride. Other studies connect fluoride use to heart disease, bone cancer, and other diseases. On the other hand, the supporters of fluoridation, while acknowledging that high doses can cause such problems, cite other studies disputing these findings when lower doses are involved.

11. The amount of fluoride found in beverages depends on the fluoride found in the water that's used in them. If it's artificially fluoridated water they'll contain about 1 mg per quart. If the water used is naturally higher in fluoride you'll get more. Teas are exceptionally high in fluoride, about 0.4 mg per cup. Today, most manufacturers of infant food use unfluoridated water for processing.

12. Many vitamins and medicines, especially tranquilizers, contain fluoride. Some medicines containing fluoride come with a warning not to use it with water if the water contains more than 0.7 ppm fluoride. If a particular medicine is high in fluoride a single dose can provide up to 5 mg.

13. Fluoridated toothpastes and mouthwashes contain large amounts of fluoride. A tube of fluoridated toothpaste can contain between 1,000 and 2,000 mg of fluoride per tube, depending on the size. Over-the-counter fluoride mouthwashes can legally contain up to 120 mg.

14. While adults swallow very little toothpaste, children between the ages of two and six swallow about 33 percent of what goes on the toothbrush, and those between seven and sixteen will swallow about 20 percent. If the toothpaste is fluoridated and a normal amount of paste is applied, the average child will swallow or absorb between 0.5 and 1 mg of fluoride per brushing.

15. Only about one-half of the fluoride ingested by adults (a larger portion by infants and children) is actually available to the body (teeth, bones, and tissues); the rest is eliminated through the feces and urine.

16. Of the thirty-one industrialized nations only six have made fluoride available to more than 20 percent of the population. In recent years, Holland, Denmark, Japan, Sweden, and West Germany have discontinued its use. Its acceptance has not been universal in other countries.

17. Although fluoride can reduce the incidence of decay it's not needed to prevent it.

With this information in hand, let's look at what each side has to say.

Profluoride

☐ Fluoridation reduces tooth decay, if ingested when the enamel is forming.

☐ Drinking fluoridated water after the teeth have erupted can also help reduce decay.

☐ The recommended dose of fluoride in drinking water is completely safe.

☐ Fluoridation offers those who can't afford the high price of dental repair, or are uneducated about prevention, a way to help protect their children against tooth decay.

Antifluoride

☐ Fluoridation of community water systems doesn't give those who don't wish to be fluoridated, for any reason, a choice.

☐ Fluoride is a highly toxic substance and fatal at higher doses.

☐ Because fluoride is found naturally in most foods and water, there is no simple way of determining how much you and your child are actually ingesting.

☐ Fluoridation, for adults and for children whose enamel has already formed, has only a negligible impact on tooth decay, and this debatable reduction isn't worth the potential side effects of fluoride.

☐ Fluoridation does nothing to protect you against the number one killer of teeth—gum disease. Although some claims have been made that mouthwashes or toothpastes containing fluoride help fight gingivitis, those claims haven't been adequately substantiated.

☐ The difference between the amount of fluoride that can be beneficial to your teeth and the amount that can cause side effects is very small. Based on a consumption of two quarts of water per day, the recommended dosage of fluoride is 1 ppm. At that dosage, fluorosis will not normally occur, whereas at the level of 2 to 4 ppm, or more, mild to severe mottling may result.

☐ If you've lost all of your teeth fluoride is completely useless.

☐ Fluoridating the water system isn't the only way to get fluoride. There are fluoridated toothpastes, mouthwashes, and bottled water, as well as topical fluoride treatments. Your dentist can also prescribe fluoride tablets and drops. These methods may not be the easiest or the least expensive way to get fluoride, but they do allow for a free choice.

☐ While fluoride has reduced the incidence of tooth decay it's not the only way to prevent it. Before the addition of fluoride to the water systems in the 1940s, millions of people prevented tooth decay through diet and/or an effective home care program. In other words, if fluoride didn't exist on our planet you could still, with the right information, tools, and desire, prevent dental disease. This fact is important to consider when you're making a decision about fluoridating yourself or your children.

Is Fluoride Safe or Isn't It?

The answer is a qualified yes and no. At some point, everything, even pure water, can be considered toxic. However, some substances are more toxic than others. I agree with the profluoride camp that at the "safe" adult daily dose of about 2 mg fluoride (two quarts of 1 ppm fluoridated water), the vast majority of people won't suffer any side effects. If that dosage could be totally controlled—if the only source of fluoride you'd receive was from the controlled water supply—I would have no problem with artificially fluoridating water. But that's not the case. Fluoride is found naturally (and unnaturally) in so many things that how much fluoride an individual will be exposed to on a daily basis is anybody's guess.

Let's say a pregnant woman, or a nursing mother, drinks two quarts of fluoridated water a day (one-half of the population drinks more than two quarts of water per day), plus juice, tea, and other beverages. Let's also say she eats vegetables high in fluoride and eats seafood daily, brushes with a fluoride toothpaste, uses a fluoride mouthwash, and is taking prescribed medication containing fluoride. She could easily be ingesting 5 mg or more of fluoride daily (over the arguably safe maximum dose). Yet no creditable person would ever suggest that a fetus, or a nursing child, should have more than 0.25 mg of fluoride daily. Our hypothetical fetus or nursing child would be exposed to much more than she should from her mother. Remember, the fetus and the nursing child both receive all their sustenance from their mother.

And what about the young child, two to six years old? Assuming he drinks only six eight-ounce glasses of fluoridated liquid in the form of water, juice, and other beverages, he'll take in 1.5 mg of fluoride. If he brushes with fluoride toothpaste twice a day (swallowing the equivalent of 2 mg of fluoride total), rinses with a mouthwash containing fluoride, and gets additional amounts from food (about 0.4 mg), it's easy to see that he could be ingesting 4 to 5 mg of fluoride per day. Yet, the recommended daily dose of fluoride in that age group is no more than 1 mg.

What about kids over fourteen and adults? The enamel has already formed, so fluoride can no longer be added to the enamel by ingesting fluoridated water. Anyone over the age of fourteen (including anyone who's lost his teeth) will be adding 1 mg fluoride to their diet if they drink only one quart of water, and about 3 mg of fluoride if they drink more than three quarts of water and other beverages containing fluoride (an active teenager or adult, on a hot summer day, could readily drink more that three quarts of water). That doesn't include fluoride from foods, toothpastes, medicines, and mouthwashes. These folks could easily be receiving 5 mg or more of fluoride daily— yet enamel formation is over.

Yes, there is a point to be made here. These hypothetical cases would certainly not be considered abnormal or excessive. Yet in every case these people would be consuming more than the maximum daily dose of fluoride. And in every case it's the artificially added fluoride that moves them out of the recommended safe range of fluoride consumption and into the potentially harmful range. Obviously, not everyone in the population actually fits into these examples, but I believe tens of millions of people do.

There's also the issue of the increased incidence of mottling in young children's teeth. Until fairly recently, the fluoride occurring naturally in water and food was pretty much the only fluoride people were exposed to. That's no longer the case, what with the advent of fluoridated water, toothpastes, mouthwashes, etc. Children in the enamel-forming stage who are drinking fluoridated water and using other fluoride products could easily be ingesting 2 to 5 mg of fluoride daily. This is within the range of fluoride that causes mottling and could easily account for the 30 percent increase in mottling seen in recent years. This important issue, which is related to the relatively recent addition of new sources of fluoride, hasn't been adequately addressed by the profluoride faction, and I think it's time it was. I believe that even though some studies have shown that fluoridated water containing 1 ppm fluoride doesn't cause fluoride toxicity, any studies that were done over fifteen years ago or that do not take into account other sources of fluoride that tens of millions of children are now exposed to should be considered invalid. Although mottling isn't life-threatening, it's still considered a toxic side effect of fluoride.

How I See It

I'm in favor of whatever will eliminate or reduce all forms of dental disease. But it concerns me that those who avidly support water fluoridation continue to say that it's 100 percent safe to continually drink water fluoridated at the recommended level. I don't believe that. Although the amount of fluoride put into a water system is rigidly controlled, *how much water an individual drinks is not controlled.* This means that the amount of fluoride a person ingests is not determined by the concentration of fluoride in the water, but by how much water that person drinks.

It also concerns me that the profluoride faction won't admit that out of the 150 million people drinking fluoridated water some

And what about fluoride's "boomerang effect"? Some fluoridated children actually increase sugar consumption and stop brushing because they figure they'll get fewer cavities no matter how much sugar they eat or how little they brush. This might be fine if decay was the only dental issue—but it isn't. What I've seen happen far too often is that the fluoridated child believes she must brush only to prevent decay, and if she doesn't get decay she's not motivated to develop a good oral hygiene program. The result is that by the time she's a teenager she'll have gum disease, and when she leaves home she'll find herself without an established oral hygiene program to fall back on. So make sure that when you begin selling your child on prevention, you let her know that taking care of her mouth isn't done just to prevent tooth decay but to prevent gum disease as well.

are bound to have a problem with a substance as toxic as fluoride, even if taken in small quantities. It concerns me that they present fluoride as if it's the most harmless substance in the world. Yet millions of people are allergic to wheat, rice, corn, pollens, and just about everything else we're exposed to—none of which are ordinarily considered toxic at all.

It concerns me, too, when I don't have a choice about what I'm eating or drinking, whatever my reason. Spinach is good for you, but I don't want anyone telling me I have to eat it everyday.

It also concerns me that so much time, energy, and money are spent on promoting and defending fluoridation as the solution to decay, when the only truly effective, and harmless, way to prevent all forms of dental disease is through education. Drinking fluoridated water won't prevent gum disease. When it comes to gum disease, you have to brush, floss, and irrigate to prevent it. Therefore, if you do what's necessary to prevent gum disease, you'll also prevent decay—even without fluoridated water.

On the other hand, while I share these concerns with many of the antifluoride faction, I'd like to see fluoridation opponents channel some of their energy into helping make effective preventive education available to everyone. It's not enough to "just say no" to fluoridation when for millions of people it's the only protection they may have against tooth decay.

I may not have all the answers, but I do have some suggestions. I believe people should be given a choice as to whether they want to be artificially fluoridated. If we started making fluoride available to everyone who wants it in the form of tablets, drops, or bottled water—although it would be more expensive and logistically more difficult to do—we would have no need to fluoridate the water system. Done in this way I believe fluoride can be a viable preventive tool.

Still, it's just an "aspirin" approach to dental disease. By this I mean that it may reduce the incidence of decay, but in spite of all the promotion, good intentions, the wishing, and the hoping, fluoride is not the solution to dental disease, especially gum disease. Prevention is the only noncontroversial, and nonhazardous, way to eliminate it.

What You Can Do

- ☐ Even if your teeth (or your child's) were exposed to fluoridated water during their formation, you need to brush and floss as much as anyone else in order to prevent gum disease.

- ☐ If you're completely against fluoridation, don't give artificially added fluoride to your child at any time or in any form. This means that if your water is fluoridated you'll have to take the time and spend the money to buy a water purification system that will remove fluoride or purchase water that doesn't contain fluoride. You'll also need to make a sincere commitment to your child's oral hygiene that includes taking care of the brushing until he can do it himself, making sure he gets regular dental checkups, and educating him about prevention. If you aren't willing to do this, I don't think you should deprive him of the decay protection of fluoride (regardless of its potential side effect), because without proper oral hygiene education, or fluoridated water, or some other form of fluoride protection, I guarantee you he'll get tooth decay.

- ☐ Start your child's dental exams early. Have the dentist use sealants on the back teeth as soon as possible after they've erupted, whether your child has been drinking fluoridated water or not.

□ Even if you're in favor of fluoridation, never give your child fluoridated toothpaste or mouthwash until you're absolutely convinced he won't swallow it. When you feel confident about this, it's still a good idea to follow the advice of many pediatric dentists and make sure the amount you put on the brush is about a third the size of a pea.

□ If you're pregnant, or a nursing mother, pay extra close attention to how much fluoride you're ingesting.

□ If you can't afford dental treatment or are unable to get involved in your child's dental education, make sure that between the ages of one and fourteen she drinks fluoridated water or adds fluoridated tablets or drops to her diet. Your dentist will be able to prescribe them for you and will explain how to use them.

While I do have concerns about fluoridating the water system, I don't have the same concerns about the use of topical fluoride treatments, fluoridated mouthwashes and toothpastes, and fluoride drops or tablets. With these forms of fluoride, you have the *freedom to choose* whether you want to use them or not use them. This means you have more control over the amount of fluoride you're exposed to. Also, if your drinking water isn't fluoridated, these are the best methods of taking advantage of fluoride.

Topical fluoride treatment If you're not opposed to fluoride I strongly recommend topical fluoride treatments at the dental office for your child—at least until he's established a sound hygiene program. Topical fluoride treatments have proven to be as much as 40 percent or more effective in reducing decay. I've no problem with having them done because they're only done periodically, they're strictly controlled, you're not taking it on a daily basis, and you have a choice. For adults with bone loss and exposed roots, topical fluoride can be a valuable adjunct to your home care program.

Fluoride mouthwash Weekly rinsing with a fluoride mouthwash has been shown to reduce decay in children from between 20 and 40 percent. As long as your child is being taught correct preventive techniques, you're not opposed to exposing her to fluoride, and she's learned not to swallow it, I see no problem with using fluoride rinses as a *adjunct* to an oral hygiene program. But if you don't include preventive education, the best you can hope to do is to reduce the incidence of one form of dental disease, decay. If your child ends up losing her teeth at fifty to gum disease, instead of at forty to decay, that's a plus—but she'll still end up losing them.

Fluoride toothpastes Nearly 90 percent of all toothpastes sold today contain fluoride. Fluoride toothpaste has been shown to reduce decay, but you shouldn't let your child use it until you're convinced he won't swallow it. If the amount of paste you put on his brush is the amount normally used, about 1 gram, and he brushes twice a day, he'll swallow about twice as much as he would get from drinking one quart of fluoridated water. If your water isn't fluoridated you might want to increase the amount of paste. If the water is fluoridated, or you're giving him fluoride tablets or drops, you may want to switch to an unfluoridated brand of paste until he learns not to swallow it.

Tablets and drops Fluoride tablets and liquid drops have been shown to reduce decay in children by as much as 40 percent if administered at least 150 days a year during the ages when the enamel is forming. School programs that provide fluoride in these forms have been established in areas where the water isn't fluoridated. As a parent you'll have a choice as to whether or not you wish your child to participate in such a program. I support any such programs as long as there is freedom of choice.

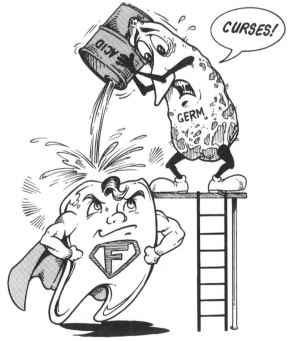

MERCURY

Like fluoride, mercury (Hg) is a very toxic substance. Like fluoride, in high enough doses or relatively small doses over a long enough period of time, it can cause a range of ailments and even death. Symptoms of mercury poisoning, when exposure is at high levels over long periods, range from vision and speech problems to depression, confusion, moderate to severe tremors, and inflamed gums. At lower levels the symptoms include fatigue, weakness, persistant headaches, minor tremors, ringing in the ears, and skin problems. On one side there are many in the dental community and various health organizations who feel that there isn't enough mercury exposure from amalgam fillings alone to pose a health hazard. On the other side is the antimercury faction, who believe that any exposure to mercury, at any level, is a health hazard, and that too many people are getting too much mercury from their fillings and other sources. That's the crux of the debate, in a small nutshell.

The silver-mercury (amalgam) filling controversy is somewhat similar to the fluoridation debate in that there are two very emotional factions. Also, just as fluoridated water is not the only source of the fluoride we ingest, the mercury in amalgam fillings isn't your only source of this heavy metal. When you add the amount of mercury you receive from fillings to the mercury you absorb from your diet and possibly your workplace, the mercury in your fillings could be the straw that breaks the camel's back. Besides constituting about 50 percent of amalgam fillings, mercury is found in food, especially in fish (tuna is the biggest contributor), shellfish, carrots, lettuce, and grains that have been exposed to mercury-containing fungicides. It's also found in medications, adhesives, preservatives, cosmetics, etc. It has many industrial uses as well, and anyone working with it, or around it, is especially at risk.

But unlike fluoridation, the mercury issue is not about freedom of choice. Fluoridation can be forced on you against your will by means of the public water system, but if you don't want a mercury filling you don't have to have one. Simple as that. And you can have the ones you do have replaced. No dentist is going to force you to have mercury fillings. He may present strong arguments for having them, and he may even refuse to treat you if you don't want them (you can always find another dentist who will), but you'll always have the final say in the matter. Therefore, although there's great debate over who's at risk, how much is toxic, and the actual role amalgam fillings play in mercury poisoning, I don't see this debate in the same light as I do the fluoride controversy.

If I Were You...

I don't believe a majority of people exposed to the mercury released from amalgam fillings are at risk, but I do believe that many people are. I can't tell you if you're at risk, and I don't think your dentist can tell you either. You can simplify things by not taking any risks and having your teeth repaired with materials that don't contain mercury, such as composites, gold, or porcelain-to-metal. Or you can consult with your doctor and have yourself tested for excess mercury (and other heavy metals, such as nickel, lead, tin, and silver) in order to determine if you're sensitive to it or your body contains unsafe levels of it.

☐ If I were you, I wouldn't have any amalgam fillings put into my mouth. Not because I know for a fact that they'd be harmful to me personally but because I don't know that they wouldn't be. If the mercury from a filling were the only heavy metal or toxic substance I'd be exposed to in my life, I'd have a different attitude toward it. But we're being exposed to more toxic substances than ever before: from the food and water we eat and drink, from the air we breathe, and from the workplace. Because of that exposure I don't feel it's in my best interests to add more of any toxic substance to my body—especially mercury, since it, like other heavy metals we're exposed to, can accumulate in the body and exhibit its symptoms at a later date. This approach is a reflection of my personal philosophy of prevention—trying to take care of whatever I don't want to happen to me before it has a chance to happen. What price peace of mind?

☐ If I were you, I would remove all the silver-mercury fillings I now have in my mouth. I wouldn't have made that statement ten years ago because until the recent improvements in composites the alternatives to amalgam fillings were either too expensive or inferior. While it's true that amalgam fillings are a little less expensive, can last longer, and resist recurrent decay better than most composites, composites are good restorations and are getting better—and they don't contain mercury.

But I'd only replace my fillings if I were concerned about mercury toxicity or if I had symptoms of heavy metal poisoning. The symptoms of mercury poisoning can be confused with the symptoms of many other diseases. So, before you run out and have your fillings removed, consult with your physician. He may recommend that you be tested for heavy metal toxicity. If you don't get tested the only way you would know if the mercury in your fillings was the cause of your symptoms would be to have them removed. Costwise, it makes more sense to have amalgam fillings replaced than to pay for the long-term treatment of any illness related to them.

☐ If I were you, I definitely wouldn't have all my mercury fillings removed at one time because unless they're removed in stages I could get a big one-time jolt of mercury. In order to remove an amalgam, the filling must be drilled out, so you're exposed to a lot of mercury-containing particles all at once. I'd either find a dentist who practices mercury-free dentistry or find one who supported my decision to remove the fillings, understood the proper way to do it, and was versed in the health problems mercury could cause. I'd make sure the dentist used a rubber *dam* (a device used to isolate one or more teeth from the rest of the mouth) when he removed the fillings in order to protect me from swallowing any of the mercury-containing particles created by the drill breaking up the filling.

☐ If I were you and I had a mouth full of amalgam fillings and worked in a job environment where I was exposed to other heavy metals, I'd get tested for heavy metal toxicity. Heavy metal poisoning can result from the accumulation of one or a combination of many heavy metals. If you have accumulations of other heavy metals, it's possible that the mercury in your fillings is just enough to put you in the toxic range. Dr. Hal Huggins' book, *It's All in Your Head* (see Suggested Reading), details every aspect of mercury poisoning and what you can do about it, including the proper way to remove amalgam fillings.

☐ If I were you and were personally concerned about mercury fillings in my mouth, I'd be even more concerned about having amalgam fillings put into my child's teeth. Emergencies are always an exception to the rule, and I'd consider not being able to afford an alternative restoration an emergency. But, as with any potentially toxic substance, children are much more vulnerable. An amount that may not affect you could cause serious and long-term side effects in a young child. Your pediatric dentist will explain the alternatives to amalgam fillings, and with the new composite materials you'll often have a viable option.

☐ If I were you, I'd check with my city or county health department and ask if they're aware of any reason to be concerned about heavy metal exposure—the use of lead in water pipes or groundwater contamination from a business or factory that's releasing heavy metals. Pin them down; don't let them skate off on the ice of ignorance. Informing the public is their job and responsibility. Don't forget, they work for you and you help pay their salaries.

DR. TOM'S TIPS

I don't believe that a majority of people are at risk for mercury or other heavy metal poisoning. But Great Nature did not provide us with a built-in gauge that we can refer to in order to get an instant readout of the heavy-metal levels in our systems. It may be that one mercury filling will be safe for most people, but what about twenty of them (many people have that many amalgams in their mouths)? It's also interesting to note that dentists who say mercury fillings in your mouth are 100 percent safe nevertheless take every precaution to avoid any contact with the leftover amalgam. All leftover amalgam particles are stored in containers and quickly disposed of.

When in Doubt

If there were irrefutable proof that mercury in amalgam fillings posed absolutely no health problems whatsoever, I'd support the heck out of these fillings, because aside from the mercury issue they're excellent fillings. But in good conscience, and in all honesty, I can't say they pose no threat. I don't believe anyone else can either.

It may be reassuring to some people to hear that some scientific studies show that the amount of mercury in fillings is harmless. But you must realize that science is not infallible. After all, it was only five hundred years ago that the greatest scientific minds said the Earth was flat, and only three hundred years ago scientists believed that the blood didn't circulate in the body. It's interesting to note that the opposition to mercury fillings is growing within the scientific and the dental communities, not shrinking, and there are a growing number of dentists who are practicing mercury-free dentistry.

But don't just take anyone's word for it. I suggest you read up on both sides of the subject and follow the beat of your own drummer. (When in doubt, check it out.)

Having said that, I want to make something absolutely clear. If you can't afford to have a decayed tooth filled with anything except amalgam, don't use your unproven fears as an excuse not to have it repaired. Later, when you can afford it, you can have the amalgam replaced with another filling. I can assure you, as long as you have not tested positive for mercury poisoning and don't have any of the symptoms, not having a decayed tooth repaired will create infinitely more problems with your health, oral function, and future finances, than the mercury in that filling will. I'd sooner trust that my body will deal with that small amount of mercury than have a part of my body eaten alive by tooth decay.

SOMETHING TO THINK ABOUT

As with the fluoride issue, there's another way to look at the mercury controversy, and that is to see it from the point of view of prevention. If you'd known how to keep your mouth free of dental disease you wouldn't now to be concerned about what kind of fillings to use—you wouldn't have any decay and you wouldn't need any repairs. That would make all these words unnecessary.

But that's not always how it works in the real world. You may have to make decisions about how to best repair decay and deal with the cost of replacing the amalgam fillings you already have. I'm confident that this chapter, and the related reading material, will help you make some of those decisions.

SUGGESTED READING

For profluoride information

The best source of information on the positions taken by those who support fluoridation and amalgam fillings is the American Dental Association. You can write them at 211 East Chicago Avenue, Chicago, IL 60611-2678.

For antifluoride information

Dr. John Yiamouyiannis. *Fluoride: The Aging Factor*. Delaware, Ohio: Health Action Press, 1993. This is the best book I've found on the effects of fluoride. You can get it at your bookstore or order it by calling 614-548-5340.

For antimercury information

Hal A. Huggins, D.D.S. *It's All in Your Head*. Life Sciences Press, 1989. You can order this book, and ask questions about your mercury concerns, by calling 800-331-2303.

Sam Ziff. *The Toxic Time Bomb*. Santa Fe, N. Mex.: Aurora Press, 1989.

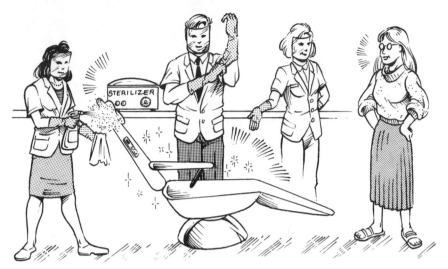

Chapter 19

AIDS, Hepatitis, and the Dental Team

AIDS (acquired immunodeficiency syndrome) is real. It is no longer someone else's problem, and you can't escape from it by hiding your head in the sand. You owe it to yourself to gather the *facts* you need to understand what AIDS is and what your chances are of acquiring AIDS at the dental office. If the information you have acquired about AIDS stems from ignorance, fear, or prejudice, and you're using it as a reason to avoid dental treatment, you don't have the right information. Going to the dentist won't increase your chance of getting AIDS. There's no reason to lose your teeth because of unfounded fears.

AIDS: THE FACTS

AIDS is caused by a virus called the *human immunodeficiency virus* (HIV). The way this virus is most commonly transmitted is through sexual contact, needle sharing, and blood transfusions involving contaminated blood and blood products. The HIV virus can also pass from mother to fetus. As of early 1994, there's no evidence that AIDS is transmitted by saliva, casual contact, or through breathing. It's important to understand this. If it were as readily transmittable as some other communicable diseases, everyone would have contracted it by now.

Being infected with the HIV virus does not mean you have AIDS. Although you may be infected, the virus may remain dormant for years. You actually have AIDS when the virus becomes active and begins to attack your immune system. AIDS doesn't kill directly. It depresses the body's immune system so that it can no longer fight off other diseases. AIDS patients die of the "secondary infections" that result—pneumonia, tuberculosis, or one of the many other diseases and infections that can kill if the body can't fight them off. Also, not everyone who is exposed to the HIV virus gets infected with the virus.

The treatment for AIDS is twofold. One approach is to fight the virus itself with any one, or a combination, of the many new anti-AIDS drugs. At the same time, the secondary diseases that show up are treated with antibiotics, antifungal drugs, and other appropriate medicines.

The above is but a brief and general description of AIDS. I suggest you write to the Centers for Disease Control, 1600 Clifton Road N.E., Atlanta, GA 30333, if you wish further, and more detailed, information. The CDC also has an AIDS hotline, 800-342-2437. You can also contact your physician or local health clinic for AIDS information.

Who's at Risk at the Dental Office

In 1993 there were over 500 million visits to the dentist. That figure includes people who went only once and those who went many times. Out of those 500 million visits, as of this writing, there have been fewer than ten cases of AIDS believed to be acquired at the dental office. Compare this figure with other statistics: hundreds of people die every year from common aspirin allergies, and hundreds of thousands die from accidents. Any way you do the math it'll come out the same—your personal risk of getting AIDS at the dental office is infinitesimally small. But however small it may be, there's still a risk, and it's still a very deadly disease.

The dentist and his staff are a thousand times more at risk for contacting AIDS than you as a patient will ever be. Every working day they're exposed to ten to thirty-plus patients. This means that they'll have instituted every disease-preventive measure known in order to protect themselves from getting AIDS from the patient. *That's very good news for you, because the same measures he takes to protect himself from you protects you from him.*

AIDS Testing

AIDS testing is important and has great value, but it's not a prevention and it's not a cure. And even if you test negative, it's not a guarantee that you won't be exposed to AIDS in the future.

The only thing that AIDS testing can do is tell you if you have AIDS or the HIV virus at the moment of the test. This could mean, if you do have AIDS or the HIV virus, that you'll be able to start treatment early. It can also provide you with peace of mind, especially if you have any reason to think you may have been exposed.

But I want to be perfectly clear about what testing *doesn't* do for you as a dental patient. Even if your dentist and his staff were periodically tested for AIDS, it wouldn't protect you from the disease. It would only show that they don't have the HIV virus at the moment the test was taken. It's no guarantee that they won't contract the virus the day after the test. In order for AIDS testing to be 100 percent effective the dental staff would have to be tested every morning before work, with instant results available. And in order to protect the dental team each patient would have to be tested before the appointment. This isn't practical, nor do the statistics indicate it's necessary (so few people have contracted AIDS from their dentist). The bottom line is that testing, as

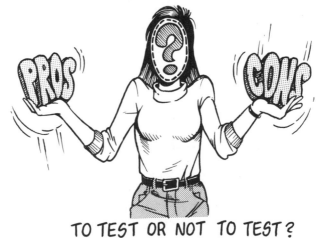

TO TEST OR NOT TO TEST?

valuable as it is, has nothing to do with protecting you from contracting AIDS in the dental office.

The ideal in this situation is for everyone to be tested and, if the test is positive, to inform anyone who may be at risk of the results. But AIDS testing isn't mandatory, and it isn't likely to become mandatory any time soon. Given that, the best way to deal with it is *prevention* and *protection*.

What's Being Done to Protect You

Many protective measures can be taken—and are being taken—to protect you from contracting AIDS at the dental office. These are very important because at this point in the war on AIDS, prevention is the only real "cure." I believe that once you are familiar with what your dentist is doing to protect you, himself, and his staff you'll feel completely confident about any visit to the dental office.

The single most important thing that is being done to protect you has to do with the dentist's own highly motivated desire to protect himself. OSHA (Occupation Safety and Health Administration) is now directly involved in establishing and enforcing strict standards for protecting employees of the dental office. These standards are extensive and thorough, and most are legally binding on the dentist. If you want to know exactly what they are, I suggest you write to OSHA, 200 Constitution Avenue, N.W., Washington, D.C. 20210. Other regulatory agencies that can also set protective guidelines for infection control at the dental office are the Environmental Protection Agency (EPA), CDC, and many state and local agencies. The American Dental Association (ADA) has also come to the forefront of the preventive movement to protect you and the dentist from AIDS and other infectious diseases. I myself would feel 100 percent safe going to any dental office that is following the procedures recommended by these agencies.

To make sure that your dentist is following the required and recommended protective procedures you can do the following:

- ☐ Ask the receptionist, the office manager, the dentist, or the hygienist if they have implemented OSHA, CDC, EPA, and ADA guidelines for preventing the transmittal of *all* infectious diseases you could be exposed to. These guidelines include the sterilization and disinfection of all instruments and equipment that come in contact with the hands or with the blood or other body fluids, including saliva. You won't always be able to see if the dental office truly complies, but do ask, then make a note of whom you asked, the date you asked, and the answers you received. Keep this information with your other dental records. Also ask if they follow the proper procedures for disposing of waste materials.

☐ Notice if the dentist, hygienist, and dental assistant(s) wear gloves, wraparound protective glasses or goggles with a protective paper or cloth face mask, or a full-face plastic shield (like the ones welders use).

☐ If they leave the room you're in and don't change their gloves in front of you when they reenter, politely ask them to do so.

☐ Ask your dentist if he has switched to the new kind of hand piece (the apparatus that holds the drill). One study has suggested that dental hand pieces can be carriers of the HIV and other viruses. Because of this, over 70 percent of dentists are now using a new type of hand piece that can be *autoclaved* (sterilized). The feeling in the profession is that it'll soon be mandatory. It is this type of legitimate questioning that can serve as a motivation for your dentist to change, if he hasn't done so already.

☐ Most dental hygienists now use disposable hand pieces when they polish teeth. Ask yours if her sterilization process complies with the required guidelines.

Protecting Yourself

Eliminating dental disease, and keeping free from it, is important to everyone. It's even more important to those with AIDS or the HIV virus. I've already told you about the added stress that gum disease places on your immune system, every minute of every day you have the disease (see Chapter 1). In my opinion gum disease overworks your immune system, which in turn lowers your resistance to AIDS as well as any other infectious disease. I also believe that those without periodontal disease have a better chance of fighting off exposure to the HIV virus. I know that if I contracted the HIV virus I'd do whatever it takes, in time and money, to have the healthiest mouth in the world and to keep it that way.

Oral Signs of AIDS

Certain oral diseases usually show up before or at the same time as other, more obvious, nonoral symptoms of AIDS. Over 50 percent of those who have AIDS or are HIV positive had specific oral complaints, such as pain around the teeth, swallowing problems, intraoral bleeding, and canker sores. Nearly 90 percent required dental treatment. Therefore, although testing for the HIV virus in your blood is certainly the definitive way to find out if you have AIDS, looking for signs of these oral diseases during your home examination can lead to early detection. (See Chapter 3.) Make sure your dentist and hygienist are looking for them too. These diseases are:

- ☐ Any form of periodontal disease, sore, or ulcer that doesn't respond to treatment
- ☐ Bone loss that is more rapid than would normally be seen with the type of periodontal disease you have
- ☐ Herpes simplex
- ☐ Candidiasis
- ☐ ANUG (acute necrotizing ulcerative gingivostomatitis)
- ☐ Kaposi's sarcoma
- ☐ Hairy leukoplakia

HEPATITIS B AND OTHER INFECTIOUS DISEASES

AIDS is not the only infectious disease you and the dental team could be exposed to at the dental office. Hepatitis B, the flu, and the common cold are among the other communicable diseases that can be contracted. In fact, you have a much greater chance of contracting the hepatitis B virus at the dental office than the HIV virus, but because more and more dentists, assistants, and hygienists are being vaccinated for hepatitis B (over 75 percent as of 1991) the incidence of this virus has been drastically reduced. Although hepatitis can be fatal, you can be vaccinated against it, and it can be successfully treated if it's caught and treated early. Until the AIDS scare, however, not every dental office did all they could to protect themselves or the patient from hepatitis. But AIDS has changed all of that. The precautions now taken to protect you and the office staff from AIDS also help to protect you from hepatitis and other infectious diseases.

The most obvious early signs of hepatitis are fever, fatigue with no obvious cause, loss of weight, nausea and vomiting, and abnormal and constant stomach aches and pains. As the disease progresses, all these symptoms increase in severity, and along with jaundice (the skin taking on a yellowish color), depression usually appears. If you have any of these symptoms (you might not get them all), you should see your doctor as soon as possible.

IN SUMMARY

I hope that you now understand that the chance of getting AIDS at the dental office is very small. In fact, the precautions taken by the dental team, in response to the AIDS epidemic, actually make going to the dentist safer than it has ever been before because they protect you against other diseases as well. If you take the time to find a dental office that is observing governmental disease-control practices, the fear of contracting AIDS will no longer be a legitimate excuse for not having your dental disease treated and repaired.

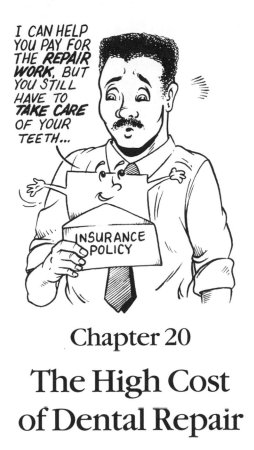

Chapter 20

The High Cost of Dental Repair

B y now you've figured out that this book isn't only about preventing dental disease and saving your teeth: it's also about motivation. If the destructiveness of dental disease, to your teeth and your overall health, has not yet motivated you to take care of your mouth, maybe the high cost dental repair will. By practicing sound oral hygiene, you'll not only save your teeth and gums, you'll also save a great deal of money and time.

Unfortunately, prevention has traditionally taken a back seat to dental repair. Most people still think that there's no way to effectively deal with dental disease, except to have their teeth repaired after the damage has been done. Then they find that they can't afford to have them repaired. In fact, the high cost of dental repair has kept tens of millions of people from seeking treatment and repair. This approach is like putting the cart before the horse.

No matter how you look at it, prevention is the only way to deal with the high cost of dentistry, now and in the future. Until prevention becomes an integral part of your holistic dental treatment plan you'll never escape from the continuous cycle of disease–repair (\$)–disease–repair (\$). Although dental repair may not be affordable to many people, *prevention* most certainly is.

Before I talk about dealing with the immediate costs of dental repair, I want to suggest a way to put the cost of neglecting your oral hygiene in a larger perspective.

ANOTHER WAY TO LOOK AT IT

Money

One way to look at dental repair is to consider what it can cost you over the long haul. According to my projections, the average cost of dental repair (excluding emergency treatment) in 1994 will be about \$400 per person. If you're twenty years old and start paying \$400 per year for dental repair and continue paying until you're seventy, you'd end up spending \$20,000. Even if you subtract hygiene therapy, exams, and the replacing of old fillings, you're looking at a substantial amount of money. And that's just the average cost. You could be one of those people whose per-year repair bill is much greater (someone has to bump up that average). Be honest, couldn't you think of something better to do with that money?

Now let's take a look at this issue from another perspective—investing what you'd save if you prevented dental disease. Using the same time frame, what if you placed \$400 per year into a savings account at 5 percent interest? You'd end up with a total return of over \$116,000 by age seventy. So what are your choices? You could be looking at \$20,000 in the red or \$116,000 in the black. What would you rather have—the dentures or the money? These numbers aren't going to be the same for everyone (you may not begin your preventive program until you're forty), but you can't fault the logic. Prevention not only saves your teeth but saves a whole lot of your money.

Time

You've heard a lot of theories about whether or not we've all been created equal. On one score at least, no one can argue: we all get twenty-four hours a day. I myself value time more than money. But, as some folks say, time is money. The bottom line is that in terms of time as well as money, prevention returns a lot for a little.

Over your lifetime, if you stay stuck in the disease–repair cycle, you'll spend at least 325 days of your valuable time at the dental office, driving to and from the dental office, and earning the money it will take to pay for your repair work. Turn the coin over, and you find it will take about 120 days of your time to prevent dental disease—that includes both hygiene therapy and home care. The net savings in time is over 200 days. I've already asked you if you couldn't think of a better way to spend your money. I feel confident you could also find better ways to utilize your time. Even if you've already used up some of those 200 days, the principle remains the same. If you only save 100 days in the future (2,400 hours)—that isn't chopped almonds.

IMMEDIATE COSTS

The longer you wait the more money dental repair will cost you, not to mention the suffering and the lost time. That's as certain as death and taxes. At 1994 prices, a one-surface filling will set you back about $80. Eventually, if left untreated, the decay will expand and result in the need for a full crown, at a cost of over $600. Or, uncared for and untreated, you could end up with a root canal, with the cost ranging from $300 to $700.

And as for gum disease, if you let it run its course, it could lead to extractions and a bridge or a partial denture. Depending on the number of teeth involved it could cost you $1,800 for a three-unit bridge (the least expensive bridge) or $3,000 or more for more extensive bridgework. Eventually, if you follow the trail of most Americans, you'll end up having at least half of your teeth extracted (45 percent of those over sixty-five have lost all their teeth). Figure an average of $75 per extraction, at a total cost of $2,400. Then comes the dentures, around $1,600 for an upper and lower. To that you must add periodic relines at about $150 per denture. Figure that they should be remade every three to five years, and you can see how being toothless can add up to a lot of money. This doesn't include the cost of emergency treatment along the way.

It doesn't take an accountant to figure out that if you don't establish a prevention program you'll end up paying tens of thousands of dollars repairing your teeth—and you could still end up losing all of them. At each stage, as dental disease progresses, it causes more and more destruction to your tooth. At each stage, as you can see, it also causes more and more damage to your bank account. The price of repair will go up each year, but the bottom line will stay the same: preventing the disease is less expensive than repairing it.

HOW WILL I PAY?

Prevention is the only cost-effective way to deal with your dental future, but you may still have to deal with immediate costs today. No matter what your financial situation, there is a workable approach you can take.

Unlimited Funds

If you've found a dentist you trust and you're able to pay for the best treatment plan your dentist offers you, follow his advice and go for it. You'll not only get the highest-quality repair available, but you'll be able to have it completed in the shortest possible time.

Limited Funds

You also want to get the highest-quality repair available, because you know that a total commitment to your oral hygiene means getting your mouth repaired as soon as possible. The only fly in the ointment is that you can't afford to do it all at once. This is the time to get creative.

Here's what to do. Speak with your dentist and tell him you want to work with him on the best way to proceed with the *best* treatment plan. Explain to him that you want the highest-quality work but might have to spread out the repair and/or the payment over time. He'll make the decision about what work needs to be done immediately and what work can be done in stages. Then talk to the receptionist, or office manager, and arrange a down payment and a future payment schedule. Realize that if your treatment involves lab work (for crowns, bridges, dentures) you may have to put more money down initially. If you have to visit a specialist (for extractions, root canal, periodontal work, etc.), you'll have to work out a separate payment plan with him or her. Find out if the dental office charges interest; that might affect how much you want to give as a down payment. If possible, avoid putting the charges on your credit card, especially if the dental office charges less interest than your credit card company. In any case, don't put off necessary treatment. You can also explore the possibilities of a bank loan or a loan from family or friends.

No Funds

If you have no funds available to pay the cost of repairing your dental disease, you'll need to be even more creative. The thing you need to do is make the maximum preventive effort possible, because you can't afford to add new costs to your existing bill. You'll also have to make a commitment to begin saving money. Then you'll have to thoroughly discuss the financial end with the dentist and the front office manager.

In any case, you absolutely must take care of any emergency situation. The dentist may just place a temporary filling to hold you until you get your finances together, but at least it will stop the decay process. Then you can make arrangements to have the rest of the work done as the treatment plan dictates and you can afford it.

If you have no money at all to pay for your dental work, don't despair. You still have options. First, check with your state and local health agencies to find out if you qualify for dental coverage. Second, ask your dentist or the local dental association if there are any free dental clinics in your area. Third, talk to your dentist. There are many dentists who will be understanding of your financial situation and willing to work with you to come up with a financial solution.

There are also many dentists who have gone out of their way to help those in financial need and gotten burned. The most effective way to convince your dentist that you're trustworthy is to show him you're taking care of your mouth and to make your payments on time. I can't speak for other dentists, but I can tell you that if I went out of my way to help a patient financially and he didn't appreciate it enough to make even minimal payments and take care of his mouth, I wouldn't work on him again.

DENTAL INSURANCE

At the time of this book's publication, in 1994, over 100 million people are covered by some form of dental insurance. Unless you can keep your mouth free of dental disease, any insurance plan is infinitely better than none at all, because anytime you can have all, or part, of your dental bill paid by someone else you are way ahead. But don't fall into the trap of thinking that just because you can afford to have the disease repaired it somehow makes it all right to continue getting the disease. If you could afford open heart surgery, would you then think it was fine to have a heart attack?

Many types of dental insurance are available. Whether it's private dental insurance or government insurance, you'll have to abide by the conditions (allowances, deductibles, choice of dentist) set by the insurance company. No matter which policy you choose, I suggest you always get the best work done, even if it means you will have to pay a little more out of pocket. One day you may lose your insurance and wish you'd taken advantage of it while you had it.

However, as good as insurance is there are a few things in the present system that I feel are detrimental to patient, dentist, and insurer alike. First, many insurance companies limit the type of repair they'll pay for. Some dentist sitting in an office hundreds of miles away decides which treatments should or should not be done on you. In some cases, this will mean that the dentist you've trusted to decide what is the best treatment plan for you won't be able to make that decision. I suggest that if your dentist feels a certain treatment is called for but the insurance company won't pay for it, you should have it done anyway, even if you have to pay for it yourself. In this situation, trust the dentist you trust.

Some types of dental insurance won't allow you to select your own dentist. However, you can usually pick from a pool of dentists, so use the criteria for finding a dentist (see Chapter 6), and if the first one doesn't work out, try another until you find the right one for you. If you're stuck with a dentist you have reservations about, keep your eyes and ears open and document everything he does. Then call your insurance company and tell them. There's a pretty good chance you're not the only patient who feels that way, and your feedback can help the company weed out the bad practitioners. I've constantly stressed the importance of finding a qualified, trustworthy dentist, and having your choices limited is a big draw-back of most dental insurance.

Many dental insurance plans don't allow more than two hygiene visits a year, which doesn't take into account the fact that many patients need more than two visits. Thus, the hygienist is limited in her efforts to provide you with an effective hygiene program because the dental office can only bill the insurance company for the two allowable visits. I've never figured out why insurance companies appear so willing to pay out thousands of dollars in repair costs when, if they allowed more for hygiene therapy and preventive education, they could save thousands of dollars for every participating patient. Unfortunately, until they see the light, you'll have to make up the hygiene difference.

Even if your insurance company doesn't cover all the hygiene appointments your hygienist suggests you need, it doesn't mean you shouldn't have them. Always go along with your hygienist's suggestions, and don't *ever* let the insurance company dictate to you when it comes to oral hygiene. If she says you need six cleanings a year, heed her advice. The small cost for additional visits will not only save your teeth, but also your money.

SELECTING A COMPANY

Insurance companies vary as to how much they'll pay per year, how much of a deductible they require, and how long you must wait before you can have restorations redone. If you receive dental insurance through your employer, you won't have much of a say about the benefits provided. But if you're an individual who's shopping for a dental insurance plan, or an employer looking for one for your company, I have a suggestion for you before you make your final decision. Call up two or three dental offices, including your own, and ask to speak to the person in charge of insurance. Tell her you're looking for the top overall insurance plan and you'd appreciate her advice. Ask her:

☐ Which company gives you the widest choice of dentists

☐ Which allows the most for hygiene therapy and preventive education

☐ Which pays the most for treatment

□ Which has the lowest deductible

□ Which gives the dentist the most leeway in determining the treatment plan

□ Which covers orthodontic treatment

□ Which company she thinks is the best all-around

I can't speak for the rest of the country, but in California and the other areas it serves, the dental insurance company offering the widest range of dental plans is Delta Dental.

GETTING HELP WITH YOUR INSURANCE

The best advice I can give you for dealing with your policy is to tell the receptionist in the dental office that you have dental insurance and ask her how to make using it easier on both of you. If you're like me you could read the policy thirty times and still not be clear about what it does and doesn't do for you. The person in charge of insurance at the dental office will know everything about it, and more, because she deals with insurance all the time, and you can ask her for help in understanding your policy. You can also call your dental insurance company and ask them.

Remember, your policy is a contract between you and the insurance company, not between you and your dentist. Don't blame your dentist if your benefits aren't all you'd like them to be because his hands are bound by the insurance company.

SOMETHING TO THINK ABOUT

Only you and your dentist know how much time and money you've spent at the dentist's office in the past, are spending now, and are likely to spend in the future—if you don't change your habits. You must also add to the ledger the inconvenience and discomfort that may accompany the treatment and repair phase.

The choice is all yours. Take care of your teeth and keep them, or don't take care of them—and lose your teeth and your money in the process.

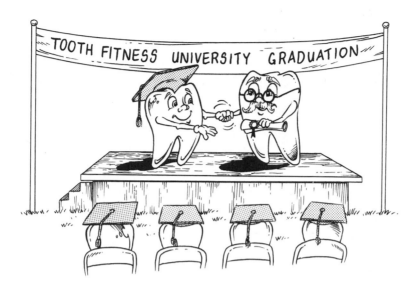

Chapter 21

Graduation

Well, you've made it through the book. I congratulate you because you've just received your bachelor's degree in preventive dental education. Remember, graduation is both an ending and a beginning—in this case the ending of dental disease in your life and the beginning of oral health. It means you've been empowered. It means you'll now have control over the health of your mouth. It means you can decide whether or not you want to keep it healthy. The information I've provided works—but only if you put it to use. Do the best you can, using the knowledge you now have to motivate yourself.

I want to thank you for sharing this journey with me, for letting me talk to you throughout these pages about a subject close to my heart. It's been fun and I wish you well.

I want to leave you with one last thought: *No one will ever care about you more than you do about yourself.*

In health,

Tom

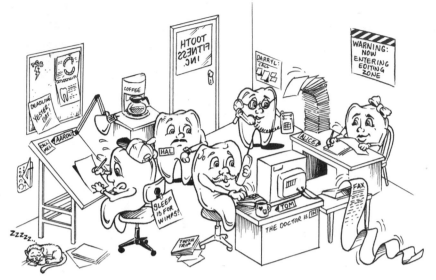

Epilogue

How the Book Came to Be

The reason this book came to be written was because there was a void in the area of preventive dentistry and it needed to be filled. You know how much Mother Nature hates voids. So she picked us to help fill this one. I say "us" because the book never would have been written if it hadn't been for the unbelievable support of some very special people. It's easy for an author to fall into the ego trap of saying, "I wrote this book," but in the case of *Tooth Fitness* if I said "I" wrote the book I'd be lying.

Writing a book, any book, isn't easy. And I didn't set out to write just any book. *Tooth Fitness* is part of a larger vision of preventive dental education that includes children's books, a newsletter, a syndicated column, and preventive dental products. My aim is to give every man, woman, and child in this country a chance to eliminate dental disease from their life. It doesn't take a whole lot of imagination to understand how much time, energy, and money was needed to undertake a project of this magnitude. No individual could ever hope accomplish such a goal alone. I can remember many times, in the beginning of the project, when I got very discouraged and felt like giving up. And each time, someone came to my rescue and offered me the moral, spiritual, or financial help needed to keep the project alive.

It would take an entire book to describe the role every individual played in making this book a reality. But they know, and I know. The words "Thank you very much" could never express the gratitude I feel. There isn't enough room on the book cover to put everyone's name alongside mine, but that doesn't mean they don't all deserve to be there.

I want to give special thanks to those who have been through the most with me. If it weren't for the support of my very best friend, Dr. Joseph Arancio, the book would never have gotten off the ground. Thanks, Joseph. Without the love and support of Lita Stone, I doubt if I could've made it through the early struggles. She helped with the editing, from a patient's point of view, and provided emotional support when I needed it the most. I want to offer special thanks to Michael, Susan, and Stephen Talerico, who appeared in my life at the perfect moment. And I want to extend my sincere gratitude to one of the nicest, most unselfish human beings on the planet, Don Gerrard. He not only made my first book a reality but was of invaluable assistance in making this one a reality.

It seemed that whenever a crisis occurred there was always someone there to help solve it. These people deserve special mention. Thanks to Hal Hershey, who so beautifully designed the book. Hal was like a beacon in a storm and guided me through some very difficult times. And then there was the editor, Alice Klein. Some people may be able to write a book without the help of an editor, but I'm not one of them. Fortunately I found Alice—for me and for you, the reader. Alice is an editor without peer, and if you like the book she deserves equal credit. (If you're seriously thinking about writing a book, the best thing I can tell you is to use Hal and Alice.)

And then there were those who not only gave their time but also their financial support. Without their help I'd still just be thinking about writing the book. Special thanks to Darryl and Karen Bouchard. Darryl devoted a year of his time to the project, and not only was his help invaluable but we became good friends. Thanks a whole lot. Heartfelt thanks to Hunter and Audie Black, who were always there when I needed them the most; to Jeff Cram, who understands what it's like to write a book and calmly helped guide me; and to Phil Jones, whose timely support helped keep the project going. Thanks to Derek and Lori Van Atta, Celestine Scott, Michael and Laura Herrman, and Richard Sanders, whose moral support was indispensable. And there's more. I doubt if I could have made it through the last stages if it weren't for the unselfish support of Alex Mendelsohn. I will forever be grateful for the peaceful, loving sanctuary she provided me during the very challenging editing process.

Dr. George Crispo and his entire staff (especially Beverly, Jan, Victoria, and Valerie) deserve a special "Thank you" for their generous support at a crucial time. And thank you to Patricia McGuire, RDH extraordinaire, who unselfishly donated her time and experience; and to Linda Jones, the book's publicist, for her continuing good work.

I know you loved the drawings, and I want to acknowledge the artist. Thanks, Aaron.

I'm acknowledging everyone else in alphabetical order for simplicity, but this in no way reflects the support I was given. Though I want to include everyone who helped in any way, I may have inadvertently left someone out—if so, I apologize. You all know how much you contributed and how important you were. Thanks to the Ananda Community; Donny and Jackie Ayers and kids; Hal Bennett; Kathleen Bowes; Leonard Charles; Dr. Bob Christoffersen; Vince and Betty Colletto; Jerry and Cathy Colletto; Beau and Virginia Connell; George and Mary Cornelius; Country Copy, Nevada City; my family; Chuck and Shirley Faxon; Joan Faxon; Dr. Steve Guerra; Jacoba; Judith Kovacs; Kathy, David, and kids (Ryan, Matty, Josh, and Kaitlin); Chic Lotz; my Macintosh II si computer; Barbara McNally; Patrick Mervin; Mickey and Anna; Stewart Miller; Lynn Milliman; Charles Muir; Debbi Olsen; Catherine Rice; Russ, Elizabeth, Sequoia, and Michael Schrieber; Shawn and Shelly; Karen, Nevile, and Floyd Silliman; Stu, Patt, and the boys; Dr. Bruce West; Pete and Irene Witcher; and Sarah Valley.

Finally, thanks to you, the reader . . . without you all there would not have been a book, and I thank you from the bottom of my heart.

Appendix

This section can play an important part in supporting your oral hygiene program. By using the space provided to write questions and notes and to keep records, you eliminate the need to memorize everything of importance you're told at the dental office. You can also keep all your dental information in one place, which is mighty handy when it comes to tracking it down. And as you, your hygienist, and your dentist customize and fine-tune your preventive program, these pages become a record of your journey to oral health, a kind of dental diary.

WRITE TO US

I'm providing you with an address because I want to hear from you. If you have any questions about the material in the book, include a self-addressed stamped envelope and I'll do my very best to provide you with an answer.

Also, we here at Tooth Fitness would like you to send the name, address, and phone number of your dentist and hygienist if they're supporters of preventive dentistry. This will allow us to pass their names on to others who seek a dental office that sees prevention as part of the patient's total treatment. If you live in the San Francisco area, I can recommend a good dentist right here and now—mine. His name is Dr. George Crispo.

We'd also like to hear your comments about the book—how you liked it, what you think we could do to make it better, and how it affected your oral health. It's always great to get feedback.

Write to us at Tooth Fitness, Inc., 12036 Nevada City Highway, Suite 190, Grass Valley, CA 95945.

THE TOOTH FITNESS DIGEST

Our commitment to preventive dentistry does not stop with the last page of *Tooth Fitness*. The effort to improve your health is always an ongoing process, and our newsletter will help keep you up-to-date on what's new in prevention and treatment. It offers oral hygiene tips from patients (be sure to let us know if you've found ways to make your oral hygiene experience a better one so we can pass them along), and from hygienists and dentists (we want your suggestions, too), along with updates on preventive products and the newest repair techniques and materials. It contains nutritional information, a children's section, and much more. In effect, the newsletter is an extension of *Tooth Fitness*. It's written in the same style and aims to keep you on top of your preventive program. So if you liked the book and want to subscribe to *The Tooth Fitness Digest*, simply call 1-800-335-7755. Turn to the last page for more details.

RECORDS OF IMPORTANCE

DENTIST

Name _____

Address _____

_____

Phone _____

NAMES OF OFFICE STAFF

Hygienist _____

Receptionist _____

Dental Assistant(s) _____

_____

Office Manager _____

DENTIST

Name _____

Address _____

_____

Phone _____

NAMES OF OFFICE STAFF

Hygienist _____

Receptionist _____

Dental Assistant(s) _____

_____

Office Manager _____

DENTIST

Name _____

Address _____

_____

Phone _____

NAMES OF OFFICE STAFF

Hygienist _____

Receptionist _____

Dental Assistant(s) _____

_____

Office Manager _____

SPECIALISTS

Name _____

Specialty _____

Address _____

_____

Phone _____

Name _____

Specialty _____

Address _____

_____

Phone _____

Name _____

Specialty _____

Address _____

_____

Phone _____

Name _____

Specialty _____

Address _____

_____

Phone _____

DENTAL INSURANCE COMPANY

Name _____

Address _____

_____

Phone _____

Policy # _____

QUESTIONS FOR THE DENTIST

QUESTIONS FOR THE DENTIST *(continued)*

TREATMENT AND REPAIR NOTES

Keep a record of the terms of the treatment plan(s) you've agreed to, including financial terms. (Be sure to date your notes in case of any future dispute.) You may also want to note such things as how long your dentist said a restoration should last, the shade selected for porcelain caps and crowns, etc.

TREATMENT AND REPAIR NOTES *(continued)*

QUESTIONS FOR THE HYGIENIST

QUESTIONS FOR THE HYGIENIST (*continued*)

SPECIFIC ORAL HYGIENE INSTRUCTIONS

SPECIFIC ORAL HYGIENE INSTRUCTIONS (*continued*)

RECOMMENDED PREVENTIVE TOOLS

TOOTHBRUSH

Manual _____

Electric _____

Size _____

Type of Bristle _____

Comments _____

_____

TOOTHPASTE

Brand _____

Comments _____

_____

FLOSS

Brand _____

Type _____

When to Use _____

Comments _____

_____

WATER IRRIGATION DEVICE

Brand _____

Setting _____

What to Add _____

Comments _____

_____

MOUTHWASH

Brand _____

Type _____

When to Use _____

Comments _____

_____

SPECIALIZED TOOLS

Bridge brush _____

Pick _____

Interproximal brush _____

Other _____

Comments _____

_____

GENERAL COMMENTS

SPECIALISTS: QUESTIONS AND NOTES

BABY'S TOOTH DIARY

BABY'S TOOTH DIARY *(continued)*

NOTES

NOTES

NOTES

Glossary

abrasion. The mechanical wearing away of tooth structure.

abscess. The formation of pus in bone or soft tissue. Usually due to an infection.

acid. A substance whose pH ranges between 0 and 6.9. Dentally speaking, acid can refer to acidic food or drink or to the chemical that results when bacteria breaks down sugar in the mouth.

aesthetic dentistry. See **cosmetic dentistry**.

amalgam. A dental filling material, composed of mercury, copper, tin, silver, and zinc, that is used to fill decayed teeth. The term also refers to the filling itself and is sometimes called a *silver* or *silver-mercury filling*.

anesthetic. A class of drugs that eliminates or reduces pain.

antibiotic. A type of drug designed to fight bacterial infections.

ANUG. The acronym for acute necrotizing ulcerative gingivostomatitis. Otherwise known as a very serious form of gum disease.

apex. The tip of the tooth's root, where blood and nerves enter the root.

appliance. Any removable dental restoration. Partial dentures are the most common dental appliance.

baby teeth. A set of temporary teeth that humans get as babies and that last until the permanent teeth come in. Also called *primary teeth, deciduous teeth*, and *milk teeth*.

bacteria (plural of *bacterium*). A type of microscopic organism that is found in soil, water, plants, and animals. Important in human beings because of their chemical and disease-causing effects. In other words, germs or bugs.

bicuspid. A two-cusped tooth found between the molar and the cuspid.

bite. The act of bringing the upper and lower teeth together. See **occlusion**.

bleaching. The technique of applying a chemical agent, usually hydrogen peroxide, to the teeth in order to whiten them.

bleeding gums. One of the most obvious indicators of gum disease.

bonding. A process by which the tooth's enamel is chemically etched in order to better attach (bond) composite filling material, veneers, or plastic.

bone. In dentistry, the upper and lower jawbone.

bone loss. The breakdown and assimilation of the bone that supports the teeth, usually caused by infection or long-term occlusal stress.

bridge. A nonremovable restoration that is used to replace lost teeth.

bruxism. The grinding, clenching, or gnashing of teeth.

calcification. The hardening of bone or teeth caused by the deposition of minerals (mineralization), mostly calcium and phosphorous.

calculus. The mineralized material that forms within plaque. Also called *tartar*.

canine tooth. Commonly called the *eye tooth* or *cuspid*. The second tooth from the big front tooth.

carbohydrate. One of the three major food classes, along with protein and fat. The refined sugars that cause tooth decay are "simple" carbohydrates.

cap. Another term for *crown*; usually referring to a crown for a front tooth.

caries. The progressive breaking down or dissolving of tooth structure. Caused by the acid produced when bacteria digest sugars. See **decay**.

cariogenic. Causing tooth decay.

cavity. A layman's term for tooth decay. Also, the dental term for the hole that is left after decay has been removed.

CEJ. The cemento-enamel junction. The place where the enamel and cementum meet.

cement. A special type of glue used to hold a filling in place. It also acts as an insulator to protect the tooth's nerve.

cementum. The very thin, bonelike structure that covers the root of the tooth. It begins where the enamel ends. In a healthy mouth it is where the periodontal ligament is attached.

clenching. The forceful holding together of the upper and lower teeth, which places stress on the ligaments that hold the teeth to the jawbone and the lower jaw to the skull.

composite. A tooth-colored filling made of plastic resin or porcelain.

consultation. An appointment with the dentist specifically to discuss treatment plan(s), scheduling, and payment plans.

contact point. The place where two teeth touch.

cosmetic dentistry. Any dental treatment or repair that improves the appearance of the teeth or mouth.

crown. The portion of a tooth that is covered by enamel. Also, a dental restoration that covers the entire tooth and restores it to its original shape.

curettage. The deep scaling of the portion of the tooth found below the gum line. Its purpose is to remove calculus and infected gum tissue.

cuspid. See **canine tooth**.

cusps. The protruding portions of a tooth's chewing surface.

decay. See **caries**.

dental floss. A thin string, made primarily of nylon, waxed or unwaxed, that can be inserted between the teeth to remove food particles.

dental hygienist. The most important person in your battle against dental disease. The hygienist cleans teeth, removes plaque, calculus, and diseased gum tissue, and acts as the patient's guide and support person in establishing his or her oral hygiene program. Also known as the RDH (registered dental hygienist) or oral hygiene therapist.

dentifrice. Paste, gel, or powder used to clean teeth.

dentin. One of the two interior portions of the tooth (the other is the pulp), covered by enamel on the crown and by cementum on the root.

denture. A removable appliance used to replace all the upper teeth, all the lower teeth, or both.

denture adhesive. Material used to hold a denture more firmly in place.

diastema. The space, either natural or artificial, between any two teeth.

D.D.S. Doctor of Dental Surgery. Degree given to dental school graduates.

dry mouth. The condition that exists when the flow of saliva is stopped.

enamel. The calcified (mineralized) portion of the tooth. It covers the crown of the tooth and is the hardest substance in the body.

endodontics. The dental speciality that deals with injuries to or diseases of the pulp, or nerve, of the tooth.

erosion. The wearing away or dissolving of any part of the tooth due to chemicals (e.g., acids).

extraction. The removal of a tooth.

explorer. A sharply pointed instrument used to detect decay, pits, calculus, or poor margins between a filling and the tooth.

fee schedule. A chart used to determine the costs of dental treatment and repair. Set by the individual dentist.

filling. Material used to fill a cavity or replace part of a tooth.

fissure. See **groove**.

floss. See **dental floss**.

flossing. Using dental floss to remove food particles from the teeth and to massage the gums.

fluoridation. The process of adding fluoride to a water system for the purpose of reducing tooth decay.

fluoride. A chemical compound used in the fluoridation of water systems and in topical applications to the teeth, in order to reduce dental decay.

fluorosis. The abnormal condition of tooth enamel caused by an excessive ingestion of fluoride during the enamel's formation. It is characterized by discoloration and possibly pits and chalky bands. Also called *mottling*.

gingiva. See **gum**.

gingival crevice. The tiny V-like space formed at the gum line where the gum meets the tooth. The gingival crevice is the entrance to the gingival sulcus, or pocket.

gingival sulcus. The space between the crown and/or root of the tooth and the gum tissue that surrounds the tooth. Also commonly called the *pocket*, or *gum pocket*.

gingivitis. An inflammation or infection of the gum tissue; the initial stage of gum disease.

groove. A cleft-like indentation on the chewing surface of the back teeth that develops when the enamel is being formed. Also called a *fissure*.

gum. The epithelial tissue that covers the jawbone that supports the teeth.

gum disease. See **periodontal disease**.

gum line. The place on the tooth where the edge of the gum meets the tooth, used as a reference point to measure the depth of the pocket.

hand piece. Hand-held instrument used to hold the dental drill.

herpes. An inflammatory viral disease of the skin, also known as cold sores or fever blisters.

hygienist. See **dental hygienist**.

hydrogen peroxide. A chemical used as an antiseptic to treat gum infection and also to bleach teeth.

impacted tooth. A tooth that does not erupt properly but instead remains partially or wholly within the bone or gum tissue.

implant. An artificial device, usually made of a metal alloy or ceramic material, that is implanted within the jawbone as a means to attach an artificial crown, denture, or bridge.

impression. A three-dimensional reproduction of a tooth, teeth, or the toothless dental arch.

incisor. One of the front four teeth.

infection. An invasion of a disease-producing agent, such as bacteria, viruses, yeasts, or parasites. Also, the result of this invasion or contamination, such as gingivitis.

inlay. A cast gold filling that is used to replace part of a tooth.

interproximal. The area between two adjacent teeth.

irrigator. See **water irrigator**.

joint. The point of contact between elements of the skeleton, e.g., between two bones.

leukoplakia. An abnormality of the mucous membranes of the mouth that appears as white irregular patches.

ligament. A fibrous, elastic connective tissue that joins bone to bone. See **periodontal ligament**.

malocclusion. A condition where the upper and lower teeth do not meet in the proper way, a "bad bite."

mandible. The lower jaw.

mastication. The act of chewing.

maxilla. The upper jaw.

mobility. How much a tooth can be moved.

model. A replica of a tooth, teeth, or jaws, made from taking an impression and casting it in plaster or plastic.

molar. The broad, multicusped back teeth, the largest in the mouth. In adults there are a total of twelve molars (including the four wisdom teeth, or third molars), three on each side of the upper and lower jaws.

mottling. See **fluorosis**.

nerve. The specialized tissue that connects the nervous system to the other organs and conveys impulses, both sensory (like smell and taste) and motor, to and from the brain and the rest of the body.

nitrous oxide. A controlled mixture of nitrogen and oxygen gases (N_2O) that is inhaled by the patient in order to decrease sensitivity to pain. Also referred to as *laughing gas.*

novocaine. A generic name for the many kinds of anesthetics used in the dental injection, such as Xylocaine, Lidocaine, or Novocain.

occlusal surface. The chewing surface of the back teeth.

occlusion. The coming together of the upper and lower teeth. Also, the relation of the upper and lower teeth; the "bite."

onlay. A gold or porcelain filling that covers one or all of the tooth's cusps.

oral surgery. The removal of teeth and the repair and treatment of other oral problems, such as tumors and fractures.

orthodontics. A specialized branch of dentistry that corrects malocclusion and restores the teeth to proper alignment and function.

overbite. A condition in which the upper teeth excessively overlap the lower teeth when the jaw is closed.

panograph X ray. A full-mouth X ray that records the teeth and the jaws on one picture. Does not require X ray film in the mouth.

partial (partial denture). A removable appliance used to replace one or more lost teeth.

pedodontics. The specialized branch of dentistry that deals solely with treating children's dental disease.

periapical. The bony area that surrounds the root tip of a tooth.

pericoronitis. An inflammation of the gum tissue around the crown of a tooth, usually the third molar.

periodontal. Relating to the tissue and bone that supports the tooth (from *peri*, meaning "around," and *odont*, "tooth").

periodontal disease. Inflammation and infection of gums, ligaments, bones, and other tissues surrounding the teeth. Gingivitis and periodontitis are the two main forms of periodontal disease. Also called *gum disease* and *pyorrhea.*

periodontal ligament. The fibrous, elastic tissue that attaches the tooth to the jawbone.

periodontal pocket. An abnormal deepening of the gingival crevice. It is caused when disease and infection destroy the ligament that attaches the gum to the tooth and the underlying bone.

periodontal surgery. A surgical procedure involving the gums and jawbone.

periodontics. The dental speciality that deals with and treats the gum tissue and bone that support the teeth.

periodontitis. Inflammation of the supporting structures of the tooth, including the gum, the periodontal ligament, and the jawbone.

permanent teeth. The thirty-two adult teeth that replace the baby, or primary, teeth. Also known as *secondary teeth*.

pit. A recessed area found on the surface of a tooth, usually where the grooves of the tooth meet. Also, a defect in the enamel of a tooth.

plaque. A film of sticky material containing saliva, food particles, and bacteria that attaches to the tooth surface both above and below the gum line. When left on the tooth it can promote gum disease and tooth decay.

pocket. See **gingival sulcus**.

pontic. An artificial tooth used in a bridge to replace a missing tooth.

premolar. Another name for *bicuspid*.

preventive dentistry. Education and treatment devoted to and concerned with preventing the development of dental disease.

prophylaxis. The cleaning of calculus, plaque, and stains from the teeth.

prosthodontics. The dental specialty dealing with the replacement of missing teeth and other oral structures.

pulp. The hollow chamber inside the crown of the tooth that contains its nerves and blood vessels and leads to the root canal.

pulpectomy. Removal of the entire contents of the pulp and root canal.

pulpitis. An often painful inflammation of the dental pulp or nerve.

pulpotomy. The removal of a portion of the tooth's pulp.

pyorrhea. See **periodontal disease**.

quadrant. Dentally, the division of the jaws into four parts. Each quadrant normally contains eight teeth.

rampant decay. Untreated decay that is found throughout the mouth.

RDH. Registered Dental Hygienist. See **dental hygienist**.

receded gums. A condition characterized by the abnormal loss of gum tissue due to infection or bone loss.

referral. When a dental patient from one office is sent to another dentist, usually a specialist, for treatment or consultation.

remineralization. The process by which minerals from saliva and other sources are added to the surface of the enamel or to the dentin. Sometimes called *recalcification*.

resorption. The breakdown and assimilation of the bone that supports the tooth, i.e., bone loss.

restoration. Any material or device used to replace lost tooth structure (filling, crown) or to replace a lost tooth or teeth (bridge, partial, denture).

retainer. A removable dental appliance, usually used in orthodontics, that maintains space between teeth or holds teeth in a fixed position until the bone solidifies around them.

ridge. The horseshoe-shaped portion of both the upper and lower jaw. It supports a denture or partial after the teeth are lost.

root. The part of the tooth below the crown, normally encased in the jawbone. It is made up of dentin, includes the root canal, and is covered by cementum.

root canal. The hollow part of the tooth's root. It runs from the tip of the root into the pulp. Also used to refer to **root canal therapy**, the process of treating disease or inflammation of the pulp or root canal. This involves removing the pulp and root nerve and filling the canal(s) with an appropriate material to permanently seal it.

root planing. The process of scaling and planing exposed root surfaces to remove all calculus, plaque, and infected tissue.

rubber dam. A thin piece of rubber material that is used to isolate one or more teeth from the rest of the mouth.

saliva. A clear, watery fluid that is secreted by the mouth's salivary glands.

scaling. A procedure used to clean the teeth.

sealant. A composite material used to seal the decay-prone pits, fissures, and grooves of both children's and adult's teeth against decay.

six-year molar. The first permanent tooth to erupt, usually between the ages of five and six.

socket. The hole in the jawbone into which the tooth fits.

space maintainer. A dental appliance that fills the space of a lost tooth or teeth and prevents the other teeth from moving into the space. Used especially in orthodontic and pediatric treatment.

stainless steel crown. A premade crown, shaped like a tooth, that is used to temporarily cover a seriously decayed or broken down tooth. Used most often on children's teeth.

stain. Any discoloration of the tooth.

subgingival scaling. The removal of calculus and plaque found below the gum line on the enamel or root.

sulcus. See **gingival sulcus**.

supragingival scaling. The removal of calculus and plaque found on the tooth above the gum line.

systemic. Relating to the whole body.

tartar. See **calculus**.

teething. The process by which erupting teeth push through the gums.

temporomandibular joint (TMJ). Where the lower jaw attaches to the skull.

third molar. The last of the three molar teeth, also called *wisdom teeth*. There are four third molars, two in the lower jaw and two in the upper jaw, one on each side. Some people are born without third molars.

tissue. In dentistry, this term usually refers to the gums, as in "gum tissue." Also refers to soft tissues of the mouth, e.g., inside of the cheeks and floor of the mouth.

TMJ syndrome. An abnormal condition of the jaw joints that usually involves pain or discomfort in the joints and ligaments that attach the lower jaw to the skull or in the muscles of mastication.

tongue thrusting. The forceful projecting, and/or holding, of the tongue against the front teeth.

tooth. One of the hard bony appendages that are borne on the jaws and are used in the biting and mastication of food. Humans normally have two sets: twenty baby teeth, followed by thirty-two permanent teeth.

toothache. Pain resulting from an irritated or infected nerve in the tooth.

topical. Relating to anything applied to the surface of the teeth, gums, or oral tissue, e.g., topical anesthetic, topical fluoride.

treatment. Any action by the dentist, the dental hygienist, or the office staff that helps to remedy a particular disease or dysfunction.

treatment plan. A list of the work the dentist proposes to perform on a dental patient based on the results of the dentist's X rays, examination, and diagnosis. Often more than one treatment plan is presented.

treatment, preventive. Any action taken by the patient, assisted by the dentist, hygienist, and the office staff that serves to prevent dental or other disease.

trench mouth. See **ANUG**.

tumor. An abnormal growth of body tissue.

veneer. An artificial filling material, usually plastic, composite, or porcelain, that is used to provide an aesthetic covering over the visible surface of a tooth. Most often used on front teeth.

Vincent's infection. See **ANUG**.

water irrigator. Any machine that uses a stream of water to remove food particles from the mouth and to stimulate and massage the gums.

wisdom teeth. See **third molar**.

X ray. A photograph that results from shooting a controlled beam of electrons onto a sensitized film. Used as an aid in diagnosing disease.

Index

Bruxism, 80, 224; and cosmetic
    dentistry, 233
Burns, 214–15

C

Calculus: formation of, 48–49, 52–
    53; and mouthwash, 109; oral
    self-examination, 65; and sa-
    liva, 85
Cantilever bridges, 243
Caps, 242
Carbohydrates, 28
Cavity, 237
CEJ. *See* Cemento-enamel junc-
    tion
Cemento-enamel junction (CEJ),
    45
Cementum, 45
Charting pockets, 171-73
Children, 270–93; baby teeth,
    275–80; and bleaching, 235;
    cosmetic dentistry, 290; costs,
    292–93; dental fear, 284, 291–
    92; diet, 268, 278, 279, 289–90;
    discolorations, 73, 74; fillings,
    241; and fluoride, 299; home
    care program, 93, 286–90; lost
    teeth, 291; and mercury, 311;
    mouth-guards, 291; occlusal
    grooves, 34–35; and orthodon-
    tics, 219; pediatric dentists,
    282–85; and periodontitis, 44;
    permanent tooth eruption,
    280–82; resources, 293;
    sealants, 290; study models,
    291; toothbrushes for, 93; tooth
    development, 271–74; and X
    rays, 190
Chronic gingivitis, 41. *See also*
    Gingivitis
Clenching, 80
Cold sensitivity. *See* Sensitivity

Coloring agents, 102
Communication, 6, 182
Complex periodontitis, 43–44
Composites, 229–30, 240–41, 310
Confinement, fear of, 199
Contact points, 35, 68; flossing,
    129
Cosmetic dentistry, 226–35;
    bleaching, 230–33; bonding,
    228–30; children, 290; finding
    a dentist, 227–28; and oral self-
    examination, 67
Costs, 321–28; amalgam fillings,
    310; bridges, 244, 323; chil-
    dren, 292–93; dentures, 323;
    fear of, 200; fillings, 239; imme-
    diate, 323–24; and insurance,
    326–28; and motivation, 321–
    23; oral hygiene therapy, 180;
    orthodontics, 220; partial den-
    tures, 245; and treatment plan,
    184, 185, 324–25
Cotton mouth. *See* Xerostomia
Crown, 45, 74
Crown restorations, 36, 237, 242–
    43. *See also* Restorations
Curettage, 174, 180
Cuts, 215

D

Dam, 310
Decay. *See* Tooth decay
Deciduous teeth, 271
Defects, 35, 50
Dental appliances. *See* Appliances
Dental appointments: timing of,
    202; use of *Tooth Fitness*, 14–16.
    See also Dental fear; Dentists;
    Registered dental hygienists
Dental assistants, 161
Dental disease: prevalence of, 3,
    37, 258; seriousness of, 21–22,

36–37. *See also* Dental disease prevention; Periodontal disease; Tooth decay

Dental disease prevention, 5–10; dentist's role in, 5–6, 8–11, 150; hygienist's role in, 6; motivation for, 17; patient's role in, 7, 15, 49–50, 113–14, 169–70, 179. *See also* Oral hygiene; Oral hygiene tools; *specific topics*

Dental fear, 3–4, 195–207; alleviating stress, 202–7; children, 284, 291–92; diverter techniques, 198, 199, 204; and motivation, 200–201; reasons for, 196; specific fears, 196–200

Dental floss, 107–8; electric devices, 97. *See also* Flossing

Dental office, 159–61

Dental records, 16, 175, 189; children, 280; pocket charts, 172–73

Dental schools, 152–54, 254–55

Dental specialists, 217–25; costs, 324–25; endodontists, 221–23; finding, 250; implants, 254–55; oral surgeons, 220–21; orthodontists, 218–20; pediatric dentists, 282–85; periodontists, 188, 223–24; prosthodontists, 224–25, 249; referrals by, 152; and second opinions, 192; and tooth extractions, 188. *See also* Cosmetic dentistry

Dental tape, 108

Dentin: and diet, 26; and discolorations, 72, 99; and fillings, 186–87; and root canals, 221

Dentists, 181–92; collaboration with, 182–84; diagnosis role, 40, 42; fear of, 196–97; finding, 149–55, 227–28, 250; and frac-

tures, 188; and lost fillings, 188; and missing teeth, 187; periodontal disease diagnosis, 40, 42; qualifications checklists for, 156–58; role in prevention, 5–6, 8–11, 150; second opinions, 191–92; and tooth decay, 33–34, 186–87; and tooth extraction, 187–88; treatment plan, 184–86, 239; and X rays, 189–91. *See also* Dental appointments; Dental specialists; *specific topics*

Dentures, 247–54; communication, 250–52; costs, 323; definition, 237; and diet, 252–54; educating others, 247–49. *See also* Partial dentures; Restorations

Detergents, 101–2

Diet, 257–69; and acute gingivitis, 42; children, 268, 278, 279, 289–90; and degenerative disease, 258–61; and dentures, 252-54; during pregnancy, 274–75; and emergencies, 212; and erosion, 77–78; fluoride in, 298; and disabled people, 141–42; importance of, 90, 257–58; and malocclusion, 71; and periodontal disease, 49; and recall program, 178; resources, 269; and tooth decay, 23, 25–26, 27–29, 32; vitamins, 262–63; and wisdom teeth, 212. *See also* Sucrose

Disabled people, 141–42

Disclosing agents, 113, 289

Discolorations: and mouthwash, 109; oral self-examination, 72–75; and toothpaste, 98–100

Diseases, oral. *See* Mouth diseases; Dental disease

Disuse, 44–45

Diverter techniques, 198

Down's syndrome, 44

Drugs: and dental fear, 205–6; and pregnancy, 275. *See also* Alcohol; Aspirin; Pain

Dry brushing, 124

Dry mouth. *See* Xerostomia

E

Electric toothbrushes, 96–97, 141

Embarrassment, 200

Emergencies, 208–16; broken teeth, 214; burns, 214–15; cuts, 215; dentist's policy, 157; facial fractures, 216; lost teeth, 291; tooth decay, 210–12; tooth extractions, 213–14; wisdom teeth, 212–13

Enamel: decay in, 26, 33; and discolorations, 72, 99; and fluoride, 295; and occlusal grooves, 34

Endodontists, 221–23

Environmental Protection Agency (EPA), 317

Erosion, 76–78

Eruption: baby teeth, 271, 275–78; permanent teeth, 280–82; wisdom teeth, 212

Explorer, 35

F

Facial fractures, 216

Facings, 243

Fear. *See* Dental fear

Fillings: classification, 237–39; decay underneath, 36; definition, 237; and flossing, 130; lost, 188; margins, 36, 139; materials,

239–42; and mercury, 308–13; oral self-examination, 75; and plaque, 50; temporary, 211, 242. *See also* Restorations

Fissures. *See* Occlusal grooves

Flavoring agents, 102

Floss holders, 108, 140

Flossing, 125–31. *See also* Dental floss; bridges, 140; children, 288; and travel, 144–45; and unnatural spaces, 68

Fluorapatite, 295

Fluoride, 294–307; and children, 288; controversy, 297, 300–305; and discolorations, 74; facts about, 297–300; functions of, 294–96; and mouthwash, 110, 299, 306–7; resources, 313; and toothpaste, 103, 288, 299, 307; what to do, 305–7

Fluorosis. *See* Mottling

Food. *See* Diet

Fractures, 75–76, 188

Full dentures. *See* Dentures

G

Gagging, 199

Gargling, 136–37

General anesthesia, 205

Germs: and periodontal disease, 47, 50; and tooth decay, 23, 24–28

Gingival crevice: brushing, 91, 93, 120–21; and plaque formation, 48, 50; toothpicking, 134–35

Gingivitis, 38, 40–42; and fluoride, 301; and gum pockets, 172; and mouthwash, 108–9; and periodontitis, 53–54. *See also* Periodontal disease

Gold fillings, 241

Grinding. *See* Bruxism

Grooves. *See* Occlusal grooves
Gum (chewing), 110–11
Gum disease. *See* Periodontal disease
Gum pockets: charting, 16, 171–73, 174–75; and plaque formation, 48, 52–53; and recall program, 177–78; and simple periodontitis, 42; and water irrigation, 132
Gums, 46–47; brushing, 118–19; and flossing, 129–30; oral self-examination, 60–65. *See also* Gum pockets; Periodontal disease
Gum surgery. *See* Periodontal surgery

H

Health history, 175–76
Heat sensitivity. *See* Sensitivity
Hepatitis B, 319–20
HIV. *See* AIDS; Human immunodeficiency virus
Home care program, 115–46; brushing, 34, 35, 41, 78, 116–25; changing habits, 142–44; checklist, 146; children, 286–90; disclosing agents, 135–36; flossing, 68, 125–31, 140, 142; and fluoride, 304; gargling, 136–37; and gingivitis, 41; disabled people, 141–42; special situations, 138–41; tongue, 137–38; toothpicks, 134–35; traveling, 144–45; water irrigation, 131–34. *See also* Oral hygiene; Oral hygiene tools
Homeopathic remedies, 277
Human immunodeficiency virus (HIV), 314. *See also* AIDS
Humectants, 101

Hydrogen peroxide: and bleaching, 231, 234; and home care program, 107, 135; and tooth eruption, 277; and wisdom teeth, 213 Hydroxyapatite, 295. *See also* Enamel
Hydroxy radical, 295
Hygienists. *See* Registered dental hygienists
Hypnosis, 202

I

Immune system problems, 95. *See also* AIDS
Impacted teeth, 212, 219
Implants, 254–56
Impressions, taking, 199, 237
Infection, 40–43, 51–54, 212–13
Inflammation, 40–43, 51–54, 212–13
Injections, 198
Insurance, 156, 326–28
Interactive Dental Prevention, 9
Interceptive orthodontics, 219
Interproximal brushes, 94
Intraoral camera, 191

J

Jackets, 242
Juvenile periodontitis, 44

L

Lemon sucking, 77
Ligament, 46, 53, 77
Lumps, 209

M

Malocclusion: and missing teeth, 187; oral self-examination, 69–70, 71–72; and orthodontics,

219–20; and periodontitis, 44. *See also* Misaligned teeth

Mandibular salivary glands, 83, 121–22

Margins, 36, 139

Massage, 204–5

Maxillary salivary glands, 83

Meditation, 202

Mercury, 308–13

Misaligned teeth: children, 282; and home care program, 138–39; and missing teeth, 187; oral self-examination, 68–69; and toothbrushes, 93. *See also* Malocclusion

Missing teeth: brushing, 93, 139; oral self-examination, 66–67, 68; replacement, 187

Motivation, 17, 166; and costs, 321–23; and dental fear, 200–201

Mottling, 298–99, 303

Mouth diseases, 86–87, 179. *See also* Dental disease

Mouth-guards, 232, 234, 291

Mouth mirror, 58–59

Mouthwash, 108–10; fluoride in, 110, 299, 306–7; irrigation with, 132–33; and toothpicks, 135

N

National Academy of Sciences, 298

National Institute of Dental Research (NIDR), 298

National Research Council, 298

Nitrous oxide, 198

Notches, 79

Numbness, 206–7. *See also* Anesthetic

Nutrition. *See* Diet

O

Occlusal grooves, 34–35

Occupational Safety and Health Administration (OSHA), 317

Odors: and emergencies, 209; and gargling, 137; and gingivitis, 41; oral self-examination, 62, 64

Office manager, 161

Oil of cloves, 210–11

Oral cancer, 86–87

Oral hygiene: and discolorations, 73; importance of, 181–82; and periodontal disease, 39, 49–50. *See also* Home care program; Registered dental hygienists

Oral hygiene tools, 89–114; baking soda, 106; dental floss, 97, 107–8; disclosing agents, 113, 289; free, 90; gum, 110–11; mouthwash, 108–10; salt, 106–7; toothpicks, 78–79, 112–13; water irrigation devices, 106, 109, 111–12. *See also* Toothbrushes; Toothpaste

Oral self-examination, 56–88; gums, 61–65; mouth diseases, 86–87; saliva, 84–85; salivary glands, 82–83; technique for, 59–61; teeth, 65–80; tongue, 80–82; tools for, 57–59

Oral surgeons, 220–21

Orthodontics, 218–20; and home care program, 93, 141

Osteoclasts, 54

P

Pacifiers, 279–80

Pain: and emergencies, 208, 209, 211, 214; fear of, 197–98, 199; and gingivitis, 41; oral self-examination, 64; and periodontal disease, 43

Panography X ray, 190–91

Papillon-Lefevre syndrome, 44

Partial dentures, 244–45; definition, 237, 249; and home care program, 140–41; and toothbrushes, 93. *See also* Restorations

Patients' rights, 150

Pediatric dentists, 282–85

Pedodontists. *See* Pediatric dentists

Periapical X ray, 189

Pericoronitis, 212

Periodontal disease, 37, 38–55; and AIDS, 318–19; and brushing, 91, 93, 94, 95, 117; causes of, 39–40; costs of, 323; development of, 45–55; and fluoride, 301, 304; and gum pockets, 172; prevalence of, 37; and salt, 106; seriousness of, 38–39, 44; and specialists, 223–24; and tooth extraction, 187–88; and toothpicking, 135; types of, 38, 40–45; and water irrigation, 111, 131, 133

Periodontal ligament. *See* Ligament

Periodontal pockets. *See* Gum pockets

Periodontal surgery, 176–77

Periodontists, 188, 223–24

Periodontitis, 38, 42–44, 53–54. *See also* Periodontal disease

Phobia centers, 201

Phobia. *See* Dental fear

Pits, 35, 50

Plaque: oral self-examination, 65; and periodontal disease, 47–49,

50–52; and sleep, 116; and sucrose, 264; and tooth decay, 33

Pockets. *See* Gum pockets

Polishing agents, 98–99

Pontics, 140, 244

Pregnancy, 274–75

Premedication, 291–92

Preservatives, 102–3

Preventive orthodontics, 219

Prices. *See* Costs

Prophylaxis, 180. *See also* Oral hygiene

Prosthodontists, 224–25, 249

Psychotherapy, 202

Pulp, 45, 74, 221–22

Pulpectomy. *See* Root canals

Pulpotomy, 285

Pumice, 100

R

RDH. *See* Registered dental hygienist

Recall program, 177–79

Receptionist, 160, 197

Registered dental hygienists (RDH), 162–80; and brushing, 118, 120; communication, 6; cost of therapy, 180; and erosion/abrasion, 76; finding, 155–56; and finding a dentist, 151–52; importance of, 169; oral hygiene therapy program, 170–76; and oral self-examination, 57; patient's role with, 166–70; and periodontal surgery, 176–77; recall program, 177–79; services performed by, 163–66; and toothbrushes, 92–93; and whitening, 100. *See also* Dental appointments

Remineralization, 296

Resources: AIDS, 315; children, 293; diet, 269; fluoride, 313

Restorations, 185–86, 236–46; crowns, 237, 242–43; definitions, 236–37; dentures, 237, 247–54, 323; filling classification, 237–39; filling materials, 239–42; partial dentures, 93, 140–41, 237, 244–45, 249. *See also* Bridges; Fillings

Rinsing, 136

Root canals, 45, 221–23; children, 285; and crowns, 223, 242

Root planing, 174, 180

Roots: and erosion/abrasion, 77; fractured, 188; and periodontal disease, 43, 45; and tooth decay, 36

S

Saccharin, 102

Saliva: and gums, 110; oral self-examination, 84–85; and periodontal disease, 49

Salivary glands, 82–83, 121–22

Salt, 106–7, 110, 132–33, 213

Sealants, 290

Seed shucking, 79

Sensitivity: and bleaching, 234; and emergencies, 210; oral self-examination, 76, 77; and periodontal disease, 43; and toothpaste, 105–6; and water irrigation, 132

Shots, 198

Simple gingivitis, 40–41. *See also* Gingivitis

Simple periodontitis, 42–43

Sodium benzoate, 102–3

Sodium lauryl sulfate, 102

Soft drinks, 77–78

Soft tissue examination, 179

Space maintainer, 285

Specialists. *See* Dental specialists

Stains. *See* Discolorations

Stippling, 61, 62

Strep throat, 137

Stress, 42. *See also* Dental fear

Subgingival plaque, 48

Sucrose: and children, 268, 279; and emergencies, 212; and periodontal disease, 49; sensitivity to, 43, 77; sources of, 263–67; and tooth decay, 23, 25, 27–29. *See also* Diet

Sugar. *See* Sucrose

Supragingival plaque, 48

Sweeteners, 102

Swelling, 41, 209. *See also* Eruption; Gingivitis

T

Tannic acid, 215

Teeth: broken/chipped, 75–76, 214; construction of, 45; discolorations, 72–75, 98–100, 109; erosion, 76–78; fractured, 188; lost, 291; oral self-examination, 65–80; spaces between, 67–68. *See also* Tooth decay; *specific topics*

Teething. *See* Eruption

Temporomandibular joint (TMJ) problems, 68, 70–72, 111, 187

Thread biting, 79

Thumb sucking, 279–80

TMJ problems. *See* Temporomandibular joint (TMJ) problems

Tobacco, 73

Tongue: cleaning, 137–38; oral self-examination, 80–82

Tonsillitis, 137

Tools. *See* Oral hygiene tools

Toothbrushes, 90–97; bristle composition, 91–92; bristle stiffness, 91; children, 287; cleaning, 94–96; electric, 96–97, 141; longevity of, 96; number of, 94; shape of, 93–94; size, 92–93. *See also* Brushing

Tooth decay, 22–36; costs of, 323; and dentist's job, 186–87; and diet, 23, 25–26, 27–29, 32; emergencies, 210–12; experiments, 29–33; oral self-examination, 75; repair of, 33–34; triad theory, 29; vs. periodontal disease, 38–39

Tooth eruption. *See* Eruption

Tooth extraction, 187–88, 213–14; costs of, 323

Tooth Fitness: methods for using, 12–18; reasons for using, 3–5, 6–7; use by dental professionals, 6, 8–11

Tooth Fitness Digest, The, 15, 333–34

Tooth movement, 64

Toothpaste, 97–106; amount of, 117; and bleaching, 100, 233; children, 287–88, 299; containers, 104; and flossing, 131; fluoride in, 103, 288, 299, 307; ingredients of, 98–103; natural, 103–4; sensitivity to, 104; for special problems, 105–6; tooth powders, 104–5. *See also* Brushing

Toothpicks, 112–13; and abrasion, 78–79; and travel, 144–45; using, 134–35

Travel, and oral hygiene, 144–45

Treatment plans, 184–86, 239, 324–25

Trench mouth. *See* Acute gingivitis

Tubules, 43, 105

V

Veneering, 228–30

Vincent's infection. *See* Acute gingivitis

Vitamins, 262–63

W

Water irrigation, 131–34; devices for, 111–12; and mouthwash, 109; and orthodontics, 141; and salt, 106

Wisdom teeth, 187; emergencies, 212–13

World Health Organization (WHO), 298

X

Xerostomia, 85

X rays, 157, 189–91; and tooth decay, 34, 36